Midwives Coping
with Loss and Grief

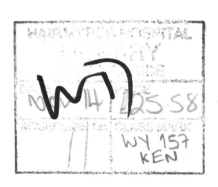

Natural Causes
By Bridget Sheeran

Could I have done anything more?
Your journey perilous, from realm to realm
Could I have done anything more?
Your perfect body and baby skin
Your gentle birth into loving arms
Could I have done anything more?
Your heartbeat strong you opened your eyes
Your finger gripped tho' chest not rise
Could I have done anything more?
Your father sang softly, only for you
Surely you heard, yet no hearty cries
Could I have done anything more?
Your tiny nose, blood filled dangers
Your mother beautiful, calling her Angel
Your features hid behind equipment pressing
Responses dim but surely present?
Could I have done anything more?
The darkened sky and rushing activities
The accusations and judgemental lingerings
The doubting colleagues and blame game torturings
The pointing the finger, the Coroners summaries
The camera lenses and flash bulbs forcing

The

pictures

of

the

midwife

Midwives Coping with Loss and Grief

STILLBIRTH, PROFESSIONAL AND PERSONAL LOSSES

DOREEN KENWORTHY

and

MAVIS KIRKHAM

Radcliffe Publishing
London • New York

Radcliffe Publishing Ltd
33–41 Dallington Street
London
EC1V 0BB
United Kingdom

www.radcliffepublishing.com

Electronic catalogue and worldwide online ordering facility.

British Library Cataloguing in Publication Data

A catalogue record for this book is available from the British Library.

ISBN-13: 978 184619 388 0

The paper used for the text pages of this book is
FSC® certified. FSC (The Forest Stewardship Council®)
is an international network to promote
responsible management of the world's forests.

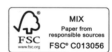

Typeset by Pindar NZ, Auckland, New Zealand
Cover designed by Andrew Magee Design
Printed and bound by TJ International, Padstow, Cornwall, UK

Contents

Foreword

It is a great honour to write a Foreword to this book. Doreen Kenworthy and Mavis Kirkham have used research to bring to life midwives' stories of being with women whose babies are stillborn or die in the early weeks following birth. These stories are sure to linger in the minds of readers, inspiring us to contemplate how we support midwives in these situations, reflecting on our attitudes, practices and systems.

The devastating experience of losing a baby for women and their families is something that, as midwives, we strive to understand in order to provide appropriate practical and emotional support. We attempt to raise our consciousness about sensitive, flexible care by sharing our stories, and through engaging with research and education activities. Over recent decades this has led to an overall improvement in the way in which care is tailored to the emotional and physical needs of the woman, within the context of her own particular circumstances. However, what is often not acknowledged or explored is the impact on midwives as we engage with the grief of others. Coping strategies can include a professional masking of feelings of devastation, the hiding of worries about culpability and the re-living in private of unresolved memories of trauma. Examples in this book demonstrate how this can have debilitating, lingering consequences for the midwife in both her personal and professional life.

Both Doreen and Mavis draw on their extensive experiences of bereavement in their role as midwives. They also share their personal experiences of loss and their motivation to explore other midwives' parallel experiences in order to better prepare and support those who face a similar interweaving of professional and personal tragedies. Doreen shares the traumatic, sudden death of her husband and hours later, her need to support her daughter as she underwent an emergency caesarean section for the birth of a premature son. She also recognises learning about loss while grappling with cancer and diminishing sight in the years spent bringing this book to fruition. Mavis identifies the significance of the stillbirth of her first child and her experiences of providing supportive care for dying family members and friends. This self-disclosure lends a poignant authenticity to the way in which they discuss their research and their recognition that we as midwives cope daily with the echoes of our personal experiences of grief and loss. Doreen and Mavis encourage us to consider how we are affected by the grief of others at a deeply personal level. By sharing these experiences we become more open, not only to the grief of others, but also, importantly, to the potential for healing and acceptance within ourselves.

Recently, I have been engaged in research that included exploring the effect on midwives of being with women who lose their babies at birth because they are taken into the care of social services. I was interviewing a social worker – a former nurse – who has extensive experience in this area. When I asked her how she thought midwives could cope with their own grief at being involved in such a tragedy, she talked about the concept, familiar to palliative care nurses, of facilitating 'a good death'. She challenged midwives to approach this situation of loss in the same way that they would approach supporting a woman with a stillborn baby – offering the same mementos and individualised rituals for the woman to say goodbye to her baby. The way in which we are able to facilitate 'a good death' can help us as we reflect on what happened and cope with our own grief.

There are examples in this book of midwives facilitating 'a good death', particularly in the chapter reporting on the experiences of independent midwives. The relationships enabled by continuity of care make it easier to engage with women and their families over what the qualities of a good death might be; these close relationships can also intensify the grief felt by the midwife. I have noted this when supporting midwives who move into providing continuity of care. This is where working in a group practice can make such a difference. Over the years, I have been in many sad and distressing situations where support from colleagues in a group practice has made all the difference to how we coped with tragedies in both our personal and professional lives. The notion of 'carrying each other' through the hard times reflects the sort of support we try to facilitate for women in crisis.

In contrast, there are harrowing stories in this book about how midwives are treated in systems where there is little or no support for them when a baby is stillborn. These insights will no doubt raise awareness and encourage us to change the design of support and education initiatives for maternity staff and all those involved in grief and loss around childbirth.

Ultimately, the message in this book is one of hope: through reflection and the sharing of experiences, midwives who have been with women whose babies have died can regain their personal strength and learn to reshape memories in ways that contribute to personal growth and understanding. Support from colleagues is crucial to this process. The challenge is to develop systems of care that maximise midwifery continuity of care and structures that enable support and reflection to be part of the ongoing culture of birthing services. Meanwhile, this book is a reminder of the need to 'look out for each other', with an increased awareness of how our personal lives impact on how we provide care in any setting and situation.

Nicky Leap RM MSc DMid
Adjunct Professor of Midwifery, Centre for Midwifery, Child & Family Health, University of Technology, Sydney, and Visiting Professor, King's College London

About the authors

Doreen Kenworthy was Senior Lecturer in Health Studies at the University of Bradford until her retirement due to ill health. She is one of the few midwives with extensive experience of research and teaching concerning loss in midwifery.

Mavis Kirkham is Emeritus Professor of Midwifery at Sheffield Hallam University. She has career-long experience of clinical midwifery and research and has published extensively.

Preface

The research here reported started as a study of the impact upon NHS midwives of their involvement with stillbirths (*see* Chapters 2–8). It broadened to include the effect of neonatal deaths so as to use, for comparative purposes, a study of independent midwives (IMs), which included their experiences of neonatal death as well as stillbirths (*see* Chapter 9). Chapter 10 discusses how midwives do and could make sense of loss around stillbirth, in the light of the data presented in the previous chapters. Over the years it took to complete our studies, we became increasingly aware of other areas in which midwives experience loss and professional grief. These wider losses and how we may respond to them are considered in Chapter 11.

The physical writing of this book was done by myself, Mavis Kirkham (MK). However, except for Chapter 9, the work presented here was done by Doreen Kenworthy (DK) and first presented in her PhD thesis (Kenworthy 2004). Doreen has been fighting breast cancer and macular eye disease and her resulting ill health and very limited sight has made it impossible for her to do the actual writing of this book. We collaborated closely throughout the writing of its many draft chapters. All credit for the data and analysis is therefore due to Doreen, any faults in the writing and the book itself are those of Mavis.

There are many people we would like to thank, not least our publishers for their patience as this unusual collaborative mode of writing took far longer than anticipated.

I would like to thank Anna Fielder for all her ideas and support, Bridget Sheeran for introducing me to dialogue, Jo Murphy-Lawless for crucial references, Trudy Stevens for first showing me the importance of reciprocity in midwifery, and Andrew Symon for permission to use the material in Chapter 9. I would also like to thank all those friends, especially Nadine Edwards, who patiently coped with the repeated postponement of other projects while this book was completed. Above all, I would like to thank Doreen for trusting me with her 'baby' and never mentioning the loss of the book she would have written if she had been well enough to write.

Doreen would like to thank her late husband, Graham, for all his support at the outset of her study, Eileen Russell Roberts for proofreading the thesis and support in placing the findings where they could be used, and Wakefield Hospice staff for their care and support as well as use of their library. She would also like to thank me, as her scribe.

We would both like to thank all the midwives we interviewed for their confidence in us and their trust that we would use their experiences usefully. We believe that midwives' voices should be heard, no matter what the circumstances, so that we can learn from them and grow professionally. We hope we have lived up to their trust in us.

CHAPTER 1

The story of the research

BACKGROUND

Research over the last two decades has informed midwives of the impact of a stillbirth on the mother, her partner and any other siblings (e.g. Boyle 1997; Mander 2006). The reaction by the midwifery profession was swift and decisive when it was criticised for not attending to the emotional as well as the physical needs of mothers who experience stillbirth. Significant time and consideration is now given to the needs of the bereaved mothers and families, which is not to say that their needs are always met. Local maternity services have protocols in place and almost all have a midwife who bears the title Bereavement Support Midwife, yet little attention has been paid – even in the literature – to the perceived impact of these losses on the attending midwife.

Many studies have identified the wide range of emotional and physical responses to loss. Responses vary with age, the nature of the relationship, the context and other significant life events, and practical implications for the continuation of the affected individual's life (Stroebe and Stroebe 1987; Jolly 1987; Worden 2003; Parkes 1996). I (DK) considered whether these theories were transferable to how a midwife might perceive a stillbirth. 'Loss' is often the term applied to experiencing a void in one's existence. If midwives experienced a professional void following a stillbirth, how was that void individually perceived? I therefore designed a study to gain insight into the experience of a group of midwives who had either delivered a stillbirth, or cared for the bereaved mother.

WHAT WE BRING TO THE STUDY

Doreen

As a midwife with many years of experience both in clinical and educational practice, I have experienced the personal joy of delivering live, healthy babies, and the paradox of the 'deafening silence' of stillbirths. I can vividly remember most of these sad experiences. If parallels between my own experience and other midwives' experiences did exist, I wanted to know what could be learned that could be used to prepare and support current and future midwives when faced with these tragedies. I therefore embarked upon this research.

At the end of the second year of this research my husband died suddenly and unexpectedly in our home due to a myocardial infarction. Only hours later I found myself being called upon to support my daughter as she underwent an emergency caesarean section to deliver her premature son, and my first grandchild. I became acutely aware, that evening, of shifting from a state of emotional shock into one of professional action. I demonstrated the human ability to refocus my mind and change my mental direction, to bracket my thoughts to deal with the here and now. I was able to function, even when traumatised, and care for my traumatised daughter.

The paramedic team that attended my husband's death was led by a former colleague and I had been supported in undertaking initial cardiac resuscitation by my neighbour who was also an experienced fire officer. During the days that followed we became constant critics of our own personal and professional competencies, and we shared our feelings of utter failure. This echoed the midwives I interviewed who described how they challenged the competency of their own midwifery practice and considered that they had failed the mother even though they personally played no part in the stillbirth outcome of the pregnancy.

My personal learning from my tragic experiences is that the grief process, as described by so many theorists over the last 20 years, is indeed a fluid and labile state. To have your sense of personal control snatched away from you, and to be forcibly detached from a person with whom you have deep attachment and investment is a most painful experience to endure. In addition, to have those complex feelings of bereavement and the joyous feelings of a new birth mixed up together is an emotional intensity that only a few people may experience. I now had experience of those emotions on a deeply personal level, and on a lesser level as a midwife delivering a stillborn infant and who is then immediately called upon to deliver a healthy baby.

On my return to teaching, I was surprised to find many of my healthcare colleagues having apparent difficulty in interacting with me, and to this day some have not recognised my widowhood. Like Lamers (1997), I found it was easier for some colleagues to rationalise that they were too busy to stop and talk about my bereavement than to confront my personal loss. Sadly, those few colleagues' attitudes seemed to confirm my emotional isolation.

My personal learning about loss, as an individual and as a doctoral student, required exploration as it was a part of my management of the emerging research tensions. Through this personal tragedy I spent long periods of time in reflection. Reflexivity in qualitative research is important as it provides the researcher with the ability to validate or seek to uphold the trustworthiness of the research findings (Finley 1998; Koch 1996).

Wilde (1992) is of the firm opinion that relevant self-disclosure by the researcher 'would seem to have an effect on the subject's view of the researcher, who becomes in the subject's eyes less of a professional and more of a human being' (241–2). This proved important, as the midwives interviewed stressed the importance of their own humanity as well as their professional status.

When seeking entry to the NHS trusts to obtain my research sample I was given permission to attend several midwifery forums. At these meetings, I took the opportunity of formally acknowledging my tragic and devastating personal loss. I considered that I had to make this statement for two main reasons. Firstly, several midwives from one of the trusts had cared for my daughter on the evening of my husband's death. Secondly, many midwives knew about my loss and might have been justifiably concerned about my ability to be objective in this study.

I resumed my research a year after my husband's death and my experience gave the exploration of the relationship between the researcher and the respondent in qualitative research a new meaning (Wilde 1992). It is my opinion that as I progressed through my own grief to a point of acceptance of my husband's death, I became aware that I was able to listen more actively to my respondents during the interviews and during the transcribing of the tapes. Personal gestures and body language exhibited during the interviews became more meaningful and, through academic supervision, I was able to work through the process of achieving research trustworthiness.

When discussing my study in meetings with midwives, I freely acknowledged my change in social position in the hope that it would lead to a degree of reciprocal exchange of experiences. I consider that my open and frank conversations with the midwives at that time not only helped me to find my road to acceptance of my loss, but also gave courage to several of the respondents to engage in this study.

I began to find the positive as well as the negative learning from my period of immersion in a state of grief. More recently I have been fighting breast cancer as many women and midwives do. I seek the positive learning from the new losses resulting from the cancer and from my very limited sight.

Mavis

My first child was stillborn as a result of malaria many years ago. I later returned to this country and trained as a midwife and only learned then the extent of self-blame amongst women who have stillbirths without a clear cause. The disease that was clearly to blame for my baby's death protected me from the corrosive self-blame I saw amongst bereaved mothers I cared for as a midwife. I became increasingly aware of self-blame amongst midwives as well as mothers and its sad effects, especially upon relationships.

During my career as a midwife I suffered a number of bereavements. I was very aware of the impact of these losses, especially the loss of my mother, upon my practice as a midwife. I was also privileged in being held in the supportive care of colleagues and clients during the last illnesses and around the deaths of several close friends. Many friends who work as midwives within the NHS have not been so privileged. Working with Ruth Deery (Deery 2003; Deery and Kirkham 2007; Hunter and Deery 2009) also made me aware of the wider difficulties of emotional labour for midwives within the NHS.

When asked to undertake the research that forms Chapter 9 of this book, I welcomed the opportunity to study the sad topic of stillbirth and neonatal death in the care of IMs. This was partly because this made it possible to look at the subject outside the context of – though clearly not uninfluenced by – the culture and practices of the NHS, which I have studied over a number of years.

RESEARCH METHODS

The main study by Doreen reported in Chapters 2–8

The research question central to this study was: 'What does it mean to be a midwife and experience delivering a stillborn baby or being party to that event?' The philosophy and research methodology known as phenomenology (Burns and Grove 1995) was considered the most appropriate, for it seeks to discover how people define reality and how their beliefs are related to their actions. Reality is therefore seen by the individual through the symbolic attachment of meanings to given situations.

Ethical approval for this study was sought and granted from the research and ethics committees that serve the University of Bradford, School of Health Studies and two NHS hospital trusts and their respective heads of midwifery services.

The opportunity to discuss the research project in-depth with senior midwives was provided by both heads of midwifery service at several midwifery supervision forums. From these meetings further opportunity to speak in-depth with the midwives at both divisional and unit level was provided and accepted. These verbal explanations were supported by an information sheet that described the origins of the study, its aims and proposed research method.

A total of 12 midwives from the first NHS trust made personal telephone contact to discuss the research further, and of those, eight midwives came forward to narrate their experiences. After the eighth interview category saturation had not been achieved, so the second NHS trust was therefore approached. A further three midwives came forward from the second NHS Trust and one came forward independently on hearing of the study. The addition of these four further narratives provided category saturation (Glaser and Strauss 1967): by then the new findings consistently replicated earlier ones.

The sample, though small, was studied in detail according to context. Data were collected via taped narratives, transcribed and theme coded. The transcripts all went back to the midwives for checking and they had the opportunity to hear their tapes. They were all given the opportunity to look at the categories that emerged from my analysis. The interviews were conducted away from the midwives' workplaces, in either their homes or mine, whichever suited them better. I sought to enable the midwives to tell the stories of the stillbirths with which they had been involved. They wanted to do this and required little prompting. Many asked to keep their transcripts, which they felt helped them gain closure on the events discussed. The details of the research methodology and method can be found in my thesis (Kenworthy 2004).

The interviews for this study were carried out in 2002. The study was first reported in 2004 (Kenworthy 2004). More recent informal discussions with NHS colleagues have raised the same themes as discussed in the data.

Data confidentiality was expressed and acknowledged through anonymity of the interviewees and security of the tapes. Each midwife was given a pseudonym.

TABLE 1.1 The NHS research sample

Name	Length of service	Clinical placement at time of interview
1 Susanna NHS Trust 1 Trained in the northern region	5+ years	Hospital-based midwife (rotational) (E Grade)
2 Kathryn NHS Trust 1 Trained in the northern region	10+ years	Community-based midwife (G Grade)
3 Ann NHS Trust 1 Trained in the northern region	10+ years	Community-based midwife (F Grade)
4 Lesley NHS Trust 1 Trained in the London region	10+ years	Community-based midwife (G Grade) Supervisor of midwives
5 Janet NHS Trust 1 Trained in the northern region	10+ years	Hospital-based midwife Antenatal day unit (G Grade)
6 Becky NHS Trust 1 Trained in the northern region	25+ years	Hospital-based midwife Supervisor of midwives (G Grade)
7 Linda NHS Trust 1 Trained in the northern region	20+ years	Community-based midwife (F Grade)
8 Claire NHS Trust 1 Trained in the southern region	Return-to-practice midwife; out of practice for 10 years. Qualified 5 years prior to leaving the profession	All incidents narrated occurred during Return to Practice programme of 12 weeks duration in 2002 at a previous NHS trust. Hospital-based at time of interview (E Grade)
9 Sally NHS Trust 2 Trained in the northern region	25+ years	Hospital-based midwife (G grade) Supervisor of midwives
10 Sonia NHS Trust 2 Trained in the London region	10+ years	Community midwife (G Grade) Supervisor of midwives
11 Andrea NHS Trust 2 Trained in the northern region	10+ years	Hospital-based midwife (E Grade)
12 Sophie University-trained in the northern region	10+ years	Community-based midwife; later became a midwife teacher within the north of England

The study of IMs by Mavis reported in Chapter 9

This study (Kirkham 2009) was carried out in 2009 to add detail to one aspect of a larger study (Symon *et al.* 2009) of birth outcomes. The main study compared the outcomes of 1462 cases booked in the care of IMs with 7214 booked in the NHS. This study examines in more detail those 15 cases, cared for by IMs, where a baby died around term. Ethics committee approval was gained as part of the main study.

Of the 15 midwives interviewed, 13 were the primary midwife in the case – who booked the woman and gave most of her care. On two occasions, two midwives, who worked in partnership and had both cared for the woman, were interviewed together. The IMs who were interviewed were given the option of seeing the transcript of their interview. Seven IMs wanted their transcript, and after they had read them a few small alterations to the text were made at their request. A first draft of the report was also sent to all respondents and their comments on that draft provided further data, some of which was included in the final report (Kirkham 2009).

Some elements of grounded theory (Glaser and Strauss 1967) were used, in that each interview was recorded, listened to several times and key themes noted before the next interview. This meant that insights from one interview could inform subsequent data collection. For instance, one midwife had done a lot of reading around the post-mortem result and knew more about the range of clinical events that could lead to that result than I did. I therefore subsequently used the interviewed prompt 'Why do you think this baby died?' where appropriate, which produced useful data on specific cases and the midwives' underlying philosophy of practice. Discussion of what the midwives learned from these cases also revealed the extent to which the IMs both supported each other and made the knowledge they gained from unusual experiences available as a resource for their colleagues.

The transcription lagged behind the interview process somewhat. When all the transcripts were available and checked by those respondents who wished to check them, I created an index of relevant factors in each case. The obvious next step would have been to succinctly describe each case, with an identifying pseudonym, create tables of the occurrence of the key factors and describe them in more detail with quotations linked, by the pseudonym, to each midwife. It had already become apparent that this was not possible for reasons of confidentiality.

With only 15 cases studied in-depth, very few IMs in practice and even fewer of them encountering stillbirths, the key factors concerning the cases, when brought together, would have clearly identified the case to a number of midwife readers. Other strategies for presenting the data therefore had to be found.

The need for confidentiality, together with the wishes of respondents, has led to individual midwives not being given identifiers. Quotations therefore are not linked to midwives by pseudonyms, but have been linked to some case information where this was felt to be useful and the midwife concerned agreed. This has inevitably led to less signposting, for the reader, of the paths that led to conclusions being drawn. However, much as I would prefer the company of the reader on this part of the research journey, the analysis must remain my responsibility alone, endorsed by feedback from respondents.

CHAPTER 2

Background

A considerable volume of literature exists on the various aspects of bereavement, grief and loss. Virtually all of this literature is directed towards providing information to help individuals cope with the emotional trauma involved in bereavement and its aftermath, or to provide healthcare professionals with a theoretical framework to help them support, understand and counsel those who grieve. As our aim is slightly different, to examine the impact of stillbirth and loss upon midwives, we have approached the literature with that aim in mind, as others have comprehensively surveyed the literature on bereavement and Mander (2006) has surveyed it for midwives with regard to childbearing.

DEATH

As well as being the end of one life, death has a significant impact upon the lives of those it touches. Like any other major life event the nature of that impact is to a large extent socially constructed. So death, like life, must be seen in the context of our society, which is highly medicalised.

Benoliel (1988) proposes that medical philosophy, education and practice exist in a dichotomy of accepting death as a natural phenomenon, while seeking to advance medical science and bow to societal pressure to save lives. Lamers (1997) writes similarly and highlights that doctors and healthcare professionals sometimes view death as a failure, a view that encourages detachment from any bond with the dying or deceased patient and their family. If this is true of death with regard to sick adults, it is particularly likely to apply to maternity care, which is primarily concerned with healthy women and new life.

Nuland (1994), a physician, writes of 'a modern death': a hospital event that is conducted away from the sight of others. Death is heralded into a neutral but cleansed area, free of any contamination and handled by experts who thus 'professionalise' the process (Clark 2000). Lawton's (2000) compelling ethnography portrays the containment of social and physical disintegration preceding death in a hospice. When death consumes the individual, the body is removed in order that it may be 'packaged' for a modern cremation or burial. In Western societies, most stillbirths occur within a hospital labour suite where the event evokes hospital policies and practices to which healthcare professionals must adhere. Nevertheless, the presence of the dead baby within the body of the living mother adds complexity to the professional processing of death. The midwife delivers 'death' to the parents and is responsible for making sure that the little body is packaged ready for removal to a mortuary.

In Nuland's (1994) opinion, death is a concept with which healthcare professionals and Western society feel ill at ease. It is a subject that we label as taboo and Nuland challenges healthcare professionals to refute this and admit that death creates within us an intense curiosity. I (DK) recollect incidents when, as a midwife, I viewed small neatly tied up packages on the labour ward or engaged in dialogue with other members of staff as to which parent the little face may resemble beneath the wrappings that hid it from view.

Glaser and Strauss (1968) have created the concept of the 'dying trajectory', thus locating dying in linear time, with a visible trajectory that we can graph. They also describe the landmarks of dying: the diagnosis; the preparation by family, staff and patient; the point when nothing more can be done to prevent the death; the final decent (of varying length); the last hours; the death watch by relatives; and the death itself. Glaser and Strauss identify the social expectations around this trajectory. They postulate that, through the acceptance and utilisation of the identified landmarks of dying, an opportunity presents itself for the healthcare professional to assist the dying individual and their grieving relatives to come to terms with the impending death and subsequent loss.

The concept of the death trajectory was very relevant to the experience of the midwives we studied. When a severely compromised fetus fails to sustain life, continuous recording of the fetal heart rate produces a similar trajectory and graph to that described by Glaser and Strauss (1968). Several midwives clearly described this process and the impact on them of observing the graph as a fetus died in utero.

Glaser and Strauss (1968) also see that the adaptation of the bereaved can be deeply affected when the death trajectory takes an unexpected nosedive, or the death is sudden and unexpected. Anticipatory grief (Marris 1974; Parkes 1996) is possible where there is a death trajectory and this can prove a helpful way of coping for the bereaved, enhancing their sense of control when the actual death occurs. Death that has not been anticipated is truly shocking.

Following a death in hospital it is either the mortuary technician or a nurse who undertakes the 'final offices' prior to the transfer of the body to a funeral director appointed by the family. The organisational tasks required for disposing of the body, once the domain of the senior member of the deceased individual's family, are now discharged to the funeral director for the payment of a fee. The professional undertaker will remove the body from the place of death and thus begin the process of 'taking charge'. After carrying out hygienic care, they will keep the body on their premises while funeral arrangements concerning either a burial or cremation are formalised.

In the case of a stillbirth, should the parents wish, all of the aforementioned would occur, except for two significant differences that are important in this study. Firstly, it is important to acknowledge that in almost all instances it is the midwife attending the birth who must face the difficult task of preparing a dead baby for first viewing by its parents. Midwives, like nurses, are encouraged to be aware of how important such a first viewing of any deceased loved one's body is for grieving relatives. Secondly, dependent on the length of time the baby has been dead within the mother's uterus, it may display signs of decomposition. Despite an extensive literature search, no evidence was found that considered the emotional experience such a professional activity engenders within midwives.

Encouraging parents to see and hold their stillborn baby was seen as good practice for many years. This was certainly the case in 2002, when the data presented in Chapters 2–8 were collected. Recent research has cast doubt upon this and clinical guidelines now suggest that this should not be a routine practice (NICE 2007), but that 'sensitive support will be required in offering this choice' (NICE 2010). Such flexible practice must help parents, but is also likely to add to the emotional complexity of the midwife's work at this difficult time.

BEREAVEMENT AND GRIEF

The word 'bereavement' is derived from the verb 'to reave', which means 'to plunder, rob or forcibly deprive'. The word 'bereft' has a wider usage linked to other losses besides death.

Lindemann's early study following a tragic fire in Boston (1944), creates the enduring concept of 'grief work': grieving as an active process. He identifies that individuals who confronted their emotional pain, isolation and alteration in their social status reached the point of acceptance of their loss sooner than the group who remain in a state of denial. From this the theory of 'delayed grief' emerged.

> If the bereavement occurs at a time when the individual is confronted with important tasks and when there is necessity for the maintaining of the morale of others, he may show little or no reaction for weeks or even much longer.
>
> (144)

Such delayed grieving is therefore likely when professional duties take precedence immediately after the death.

Stages of bereavement have been delineated by several authors. Engel (1961) describes grief as being capable of distorting both the physical and psychological equilibrium to an extent that healing of both the body and mind are required. He sees mourning as a process that should not be forcibly rushed lest inadequate healing take place. The characteristics of grief are described by Engel as: shock and disbelief, developing awareness, restitution, resolving the loss, idealisation and outcome. Kubler-Ross' (1970) stages of grieving were derived from her study of people facing death. They are: denial or isolation, confusion or anger, bargaining, depression and acceptance. These stages can be useful concepts, but they should not be prescriptive. The analogy with healing and the different time required by different people is echoed by later authors. The fundamental nature of grief, according to Worden (2003) and Parkes (2002, 2006), for example, is a fluid and labile emotional state that can be classified under four distinctive headings that embrace feelings, physical sensations and cognitive and behavioural manifestations.

Later theorists emphasise the social and cultural context of grief and bereavement (e.g. Corr, Nabe and Corr 1997; Prior 2000). The recognition of cognitive, social and cultural dimensions of grief as well as its emotional dimension led to the development of the dual process model (Stroebe and Schut 1999).

> Diversion from feelings, which had previously been seen as avoidance and/or pathological, is now embraced within a broader definition of grief and viewed as part of the mechanism of adjustment.
>
> (Machin 2009: 44)

Dual process theory embraces the variation between individuals in their progress through the process of grieving and their tendency to oscillate and hesitate between those stages (Parkes 1996; Stroebe and Schut 1999). This oscillation is seen as movement between the more 'feminine' or passive style of grieving and a more active or 'masculine' style. The nature of grief, rather than containing a dichotomy between active and passive gender styles, is seen more as a dialectic between coping by facing feelings and coping by dealing with the ongoing demands of life (Mander 2006: 7). Greene (2002) sees such oscillation as a self-righting mechanism that promotes resilience and adaptation to loss.

Attachment theory underpins much writing on bereavement. Childhood experience of attachment (Bowlby 1973) is seen to influence the sense of security or vulnerability through which people see their world and the resilience of their emotional resources in the face of loss (Parkes 2006; Marris 1996). Recognising the power of secure relationships to 'act as a catalyst' in successful coping with change, Machin stresses that 'the primary consideration for practitioners is to replicate that security in the context of their care-giving' (2009: 53). Whether practitioners are likely to have experienced such security within their professional experience is not explored. It is often expected that midwives facilitate for their clients positive experiences of which they have no professional experience themselves (Kirkham 2010). There is a real need for safe structures within which midwives can develop such skills (e.g. Jones 2000). Without the security within which loss can be considered and coping skills developed, resentment about the past, however well justified, can accumulate and become chronic and corrosive in its affect on the mental health of the healthcare practitioner (Thomas 1998).

A new term within the vocabulary of grief and bereavement was brought forward in *Death and Trauma, the traumatology of grieving* (Figley, Bride and Mazza 1997). Thus, individuals may be emotionally traumatised by a loss to which others, given the same loss, may have psychologically adapted. This concept fits well with the knowledge of midwives that some births classified as clinically normal may be experienced by the mother as traumatic and on occasion a birth with many complications can be experienced as enabling.

The concept of trauma with regard to maternal attitudes to miscarriages is explained more fully by Speckard (1997). Miscarriage is a common occurrence, which some would even class as mundane. However, Speckard's analysis identifies that while female respondents did not see all losses as psychologically traumatic events, some mothers and even some fathers experienced profound loss, whatever the gestation of their miscarriage. Social attitudes are changing in this regard, which is likely to help many women who display, after miscarriage, the emotions and attitudes that are found in the theories of bereavement already described. Some women will receive adequate support and permission to grieve for their loss. While other women may be subjected to chastisement by relatives or other individuals for seeking to grieve over that perceived as a non-entity, and as such denied support and compassion.

Figley, Bride and Mazza (1997) warn healthcare professionals against attaching their own beliefs and values to any situations that they may term as mundane, everyday occurrences in their professional practices, since

> individual meanings attached to events and circumstances, as they are experientially and psychologically mediated, are in fact the actual driving force behind the psychological trauma response and determine whether or not an event is experienced as traumatic.
>
> (69)

Lomas (2005) identifies the danger of this process within health professionals, who can approach such situations judgementally rather than empathetically, especially when their approach is reinforced by professional knowledge.

> We should try to avoid the danger of failing to accept tragedy in the lives of our patients by adhering to formulae which play it down.
>
> (52)

Formulae may be used as armour against the impact of death upon those who work with it, as Speckard (1997) observes with regard to miscarriage.

Clearly, there is a trajectory of grief beyond the trajectory of death. The grieving trajectory can be seen as a journey (Machin 2009), or the recreation of the disrupted life story of the bereaved. However portrayed, grief is a very individual experience. While every loss is unique and will be witnessed in a unique way by all who observe it, understanding the nature of loss should help in both coping with it and supporting others.

FACETS OF LOSS

Describing bereavement as an activity suggests that it is a fluid and labile entity that may be experienced not only through death, but also through other significant loss to the individual concerned.

> One's response to loss is not just emotional. Grief is broader, more complex, and more deep-seated than this definition would suggest.
>
> (Corr, Nabe and Corr 1997: 169)

Loss creates emotional pain but that pain and the grief work it engenders takes place in a social context.

Mander (2006) writes of 'the fact of loss through death' and she suggests that the emphasis should be on the fact rather than the death (3). This opens the way to examining what has been lost for the surviving individual. After the death of an adult, we lose the relationship we had with that person and all it means for us. A stillbirth robs the parents of their hopes and plans for a different future with a central new relationship and creates the tragic need to 'dismantle the future' (McCracken 2009: 63). For a midwife, the fact of stillbirth can rob her of her professional role and skills, which are focused upon new life.

Marris (1996) sees grief as 'a reaction to the disintegration of the whole struc-ture of meaning' dependent upon a relationship (47). Such meanings are personal: family members lose relationships of personal significance; attending professionals may lose vocational meaning where their professional identity is linked with life not death. The bereaved work through their grief by 'retrieving, consolidating and trans-forming' that meaning (47), which may be 'almost obsessively important' after the loss (47–8). Marris sees recovery from loss as dependent on 'restoring the continuity of meaning', a process which differs for individuals and their meanings in terms of its nature and the time it takes (48). This approach is particularly insightful in regard to the very different losses of meaning people experience following death and other threats to their ability to make sense of their altered situation.

'Restoring the continuity of meaning' after loss is difficult because of the complex-ity of meaning as well as the pain of loss (Marris 1996: 48). Meanings have many facets and are negotiated and this negotiation implies power. 'Power', as Max Weber (1968) defines it, 'is the probability that an actor within a social relationship will be in a position to carry out his [sic] own will, regardless of the basis on which that probability exists' (15–16). Many people lack power because of their social position, lack of support or because they are employees in hierarchical structures that displace the burden of uncertainty down the hierarchy (Marris 1996: 90). This has relevance for both midwives as employees and parents as patients.

There is clearly a close link between restoring the continuity of professional meaning after loss and occupational stress.

First, the main issue for a stressful workplace is not simply the level of psychological demands, but the balance between demands and control. Second, work will be stressful if there is a lack of balance between effort and rewards.

(Marmot 2004: 125)

The rewards of work for midwives include their salary and the status of the job, but greater rewards are obtained from their relationships with clients and having the autonomy to give the sort of clinical care that they see as important (Kirkham, Morgan and Davies 2006: 91). Thus, coping with loss and stress at work is very closely linked with issues of control and autonomy.

THE IMPACT OF DEATH ON HEALTHCARE PROFESSIONALS

In the United Kingdom most deaths occur within institutions. Every nurse and mid-wife will have to cope with death in the course of their professional career.

The literature that seeks to understand the impact of death on a practising mid-wife is sparse. This may be due in part to acceptance that midwifery is linked to new life and not death. Midwives do not deal with infant loss on a daily basis and therefore the notion of death saturation may not be seen as applicable. The impact of death on nurses has attracted a much larger degree of reflection and research. The majority of these studies are on nurses who practice within areas where death is frequently anticipated and an accepted part of professional care (e.g. Cutler 1998; Casey 1991; Spencer 1994; Payne 2001; McVicar 2003).

The death of a patient can impact in varying degrees on those who have been involved in caring for them (Payne 2001; McVicar 2003). This varying impact is seen to be dependent on the attachment or 'connectedness' of the nurse with the patient and their families, the nurse's individual coping strategies and the availability of sup-portive relationships with colleagues (Payne 2001; McVicar 2003).

Cutler's (1998) study shows nurses grieving the loss of some, albeit not all, of their patients. They described feelings of attachment to certain patients and gave evidence of reciprocated feelings being outwardly expressed to them by the patients or their relatives. The feelings of grief appeared to be more intense when the nurse had provided care for some considerable time and, most importantly, if they con-sidered that the patient had a 'degree of consciousness' so that a relationship with them was possible.

Grieving the loss seems to be a reaction to the breaking of bonds or attachment with the patient . . . the implications of this must be given serious consideration.

(Cutler 1998: 194)

Payne (2001) supports Cutler's findings and identifies not only the death of a patient as being stressful, but also inadequate preparation of staff for death events, work-load and conflict with doctors and other nurses as being determinate factors for low staff morale.

Spencer's (1994) study into how intensive care nurses deal with personal grief following the death of a patient, identified similar determinate factors. A correlation existed between being the nurse named as responsible for that patient's care and how well the nurse knew the patients and their family, and the degree of involvement the respondents had in the patient's total care. Likewise, the respondents described initial feelings of sadness, anger, guilt and shock at the death of the patient, while others also reported a sense of personal relief that death had ended what they considered an unsatisfactory existence.

The literature that uses the words 'nurse's grief' (Saunders and Valente 1994; Spencer 1994; Rashotte, Fothergill-Bourbonnais and Chamberlain 1997; Cutler 1998; Wakefield 2000) is at odds with the theoretical concept described as 'acute grief' that is often measured in months and years (Parkes and Weiss 1983; Parkes 1996). The nursing literature does not record how long the respondents experienced negative emotions, or how the pressures of clinical work are likely to produce delayed grieving. The greater the delay in grieving, the more difficult it is likely to be for others to find such grief acceptable. Such 'disenfranchised grief' (Doka 2001) can be lonely, isolating and difficult to cope with.

Cutler (1998) highlights the possibility of some nurses having unresolved grief that results in their inability to give emotionally and as such makes them emotionally unavailable; this is categorised as 'opting out'. There is an inference that a nurse's ability to opt out emotionally is linked to their degree of seniority. Cutler (1998) and Crookes (1996) have comparative data that identifies links between the themes of opting out and the need to be seen as coping amongst junior staff nurses. Junior staff nurses usually had little opportunity to opt out of any task they were delegated and quickly assumed coping strategies.

Cutler (1998) and Crookes (1996) query whether senior nurses are mindful of the burden that they sometimes place on junior colleagues, arguing for a balance between the gaining of nursing experience against emotional overload or grief saturation. They found little evidence that junior nurses were being encouraged to opt out as and when necessary; indeed, they reported being made to feel that such a decision was ethically unacceptable. Frequent 'opting in' is not without consequence and Cutler (1998) and Spencer (1994) are of the opinion that death cannot be equalled in its ability to place emotional pain and distress on a nurse.

Saunders and Valente (1994) identify that nurses have difficulty realigning relationships with colleagues and coping with their own emotions if they are experiencing personal and professional conflict around a patient's death.

Research undertaken by Price and Murphy (1985), Defey (1995), Payne (2001) and McVicar (2003) describe how grief saturation and unresolved emotional issues around patient deaths, and conflict with colleagues were several factors that resulted in nurse resignations and requests for internal transfer to other clinical areas. Professional bereavement, according to Saunders and Valente (1994), Payne (2001) and McVicar (2003), is a well-established threat to the individual's health and social life as well as their professional performance.

It is suggested that the degree of unresolved grief in nurses is greatly underestimated and Wakefield (2000) compares it to a 'powder keg' waiting to blow up, especially for those nurses who have spent a long time caring for individuals prior to death. Wakefield (2000) is of the belief that the distressing nature of some deaths results in nurses distancing themselves through various psychological defence mechanisms. Nurses dealing with bereavement often do so from a position of disenfranchised grief, or grief which is not socially acknowledged. It is perceived that nurses may sometimes hide and suppress their own emotions for fear of professional disapproval; the complication of this, over extended time, is the danger of exhibiting 'compassion fatigue'. Parkes (2006) describes 'excessive' avoidance of grief as pathological.

Wakefield (2000), Cutler (1998) and Lamers (1997) all hypothesise that some nurses view particular deaths as professional failures, and attempts may be made to deal with the situations by distancing themselves through a process of psychological withdrawal to a position of functioning in a state of numbness.

Wakefield (2000) concludes with the recommendation that nurses accept that they are first and foremost individuals with emotions, beliefs and values just like anyone else. Being a professional nurse is secondary, and as such they must use opportunities to explore the issues that death may cause. This acceptance will require a paradigm shift, and nurses will require help to achieve such a shift through the availability of clinical supervision or a closure conference on encounters with death. The requirement to be able to vocalise feelings and thoughts through a supportive framework is, in Wakefield's experience, rarely made available to nurses other than those working in hospices. Wakefield recognises that, unless that paradigm shift is visibly encouraged, the unsatisfactory status quo will prevail.

Saunders and Valente (1994) found that, given education on the theories of loss and grief and awareness of the tasks of mourning, nurses were enabled to produce self-initiated coping strategies. They also identify that the success of self-initiated coping strategies is seen to increase when the nurse considers that the patient had a 'good death' and that they have given quality nursing care in the time prior to that death.

Many of the factors explored with regard to nurses' grief appear to us likely to have parallels in midwifery. The parallel literature that there is supports this. Hockey (1989) found that nurses caring for dying adults experienced stress when they were unable to provide the care they felt was necessary, due to constraints on their time. Mander (2006) reports the same findings for midwives, who were unable to spend sufficient time with grieving mothers. Disenfranchised grief, which may appear in a subsequent pregnancy after a pregnancy loss (Wood and Quenby 2010), may have its parallel in the experience of midwives when they have professional experiences similar to those that caused them grief and are still painful.

It seems clear that the grief experienced by those caring for the bereaved mother can have an impact upon the support offered to her and to future mothers in coming to terms with their loss.

Marris (1996) concludes that studies of bereavement and loss suggest four kinds of conditions that influence whether the individual will be able to work through their loss. Firstly, childhood experiences of attachment influence the degree of security and vulnerability with which the adult approaches their world and thereby their under-lying emotional response to loss. Secondly,

> [t]he more conflicted, doubtful or unresolved the meaning of what has been lost, the harder it is likely to be to reconstitute the meaning in a way which successfully disengages emotion and purpose from irretrievable circumstances.
>
> (120)

Thirdly, the more sudden and unexpected the loss, the more traumatically threat-ened the whole structure of the individual's meaning and future will be. Fourthly, events and relationships after the loss can support or frustrate recovery. These four influences have tremendous implications for midwifery.

CHAPTER 3

Stained glass windows: stillbirth memories and their impact on midwives

The 12 NHS midwives in this study are described in Table 1.1 of Chapter 1 (p. 5). All of them spoke of one or more stillbirths as events that were deeply meaningful for them, resulting in them experiencing highly negative emotions and, in some instances, deep, unjustified feelings of culpability.

Many of the memories of stillbirths were recounted by the midwives in the form of pictures. These pictures brought to mind stained glass windows in that they depicted events as simple and poignant pictures or as complex images that required the observer to understand their context. In both cases, deeper observation reveals that the image that constitutes the window consists of many different colours and shapes, carefully pieced together to create the whole. Such pieces of work are unique, for within each creation there are also the beliefs, values and personality of the artisan who created the image. We seek here to present these windows to other midwives for their illumination.

For all the 12 midwives, with their differing personalities and experiences of life, it was not just the sight of the stillborn baby that registered the event as being meaningful, it was the web of relationships around that event and the meanings attributed to them. These events, with their unique and intricate complexities, left deep-rooted memories and associated feelings. Some of the midwives could identify positive learning gained from being party to those tragedies. Some had not had the opportunity to process their experiences in this way; for them the experiences were still painful scars.

THE MEMORIES STAY WITH YOU: THE IMAGE AND THE SELF

Memory is crucial to human life. Memories stay with us of events and people that have created our individual life scripts and our own stained glass windows. Unhappy memories that are linked to tragic or sad events may, when recalled, reactivate the emotions experienced at that time (Parkes 1996). Figley, Bride and Mazza (1997) explain that during a traumatic event there are multiple visual and perceptual experiences that remain within our memory. In the case of Janet, two primary triggers evoked strong negative memories: firstly, pink bonnets and secondly, a specific room. The emotional meaning that had become embedded in that event resurfaced even before she commenced her narration and again within minutes of starting her recollection.

> *Baby bonnets . . . it sounds silly but for a long time I couldn't look at a pink bonnet because it upset me, even though it's all those years ago . . . So, before I came to you I cried then!* (Starts to cry again.) *. . . that room, it still reminds me of that family* (tape is turned off, respondent is crying).
>
> Janet

For Linda, sad memories were linked with seeing a priest on the labour ward. In normal circumstances, the priest visits newly delivered mothers and babies on the postnatal wards, though imams can be called to labour suites to bless the living newborn. Priests may visit a premature or an ill baby on the neonatal special care unit regularly if requested or may undertake a baptism. There are few reasons why a chaplain would visit a labour ward, except for a stillbirth.

> *When I see a priest I really do cry . . . you see it was the priest, a male student and myself – not even the parents there, they didn't come in. The priest christened the baby in the labour ward . . . I looked at the male nurse he was sort of near to tears but . . .* (starts to cry, tape is turned off) *. . . it was so awful. What a picture!*
>
> Linda

These accounts are rooted in time, space, bodily concerns, and relation to self. A commonality emerges in that the passage of time does not diminish the clarity of the memory.

> *One was about 20 years ago . . . I remember going to France for my holiday afterwards . . . it was all spoilt. I'm 52 now, been at it for 30 years and I mean there's been lots but two horrors stick in my mind . . . another one was about 20 years ago. I had just returned from maternity leave and I was on night duty.*
>
> Becky

> *It's about six or seven years ago, I can remember the room that she was in . . . this lady . . . yes the room she was in.*
>
> Janet

It was many years ago, it turned out to be a twin pregnancy . . . I can recall the room, the registrar, the shift I was on, and all that was said . . . there was nothing we could do . . . that probably upset me even more . . . twins . . . two little boys.

Susanna

Stillbirths are always with you . . . I had just qualified in London and I was doing agency work at the time.

Sally

One was 30 years ago, I was doing nights and my daughter was 4 years old . . . and I remember walking into her room and thinking 'I can't believe this'.

Sally

Andrea's breathing pattern visibly altered during her narrative, in particular when she spoke of the impact on her.

The first event that I wish to talk about was . . . over 5 years ago but when I think about the actual event it only seems like yesterday. I can remember it so clearly and the impact the event had on me . . . it was awful (appears to catch her breath and then takes a deep breath).

Andrea

Memories are essentially a mental form of record keeping and this is a crucial skill that a practising midwife must exercise at the highest level of competency. Midwives are taught the importance of recording events in detail: time, place, individuals present, conversations and instructions given, and outcomes (NMC 2008). Several of the stillbirth narratives occurred years previously, others more recently, but the element of the precise time, its importance, and relevance is constant throughout these experiences. When a sudden and unexpected tragedy occurs, the time of day and place is highlighted and becomes a significant part of the phenomenon (Moustakas 1994).

You don't forget . . . you relive it so many times . . . twenty-one-fifty-five pm . . . it happened, yes, exactly at that time. You go over the event so many times, reliving it all of the time.

Claire

I remember one day in a matter of five minutes we had two ladies who had lost their babies . . . one at twelve o'clock . . . and . . . one at five past twelve.

Ann

It was the summer of 1998 . . . they took her off the monitor, while this was happening, they repeated the bloods, put her back on the monitor . . . then suddenly at 2pm there was no heart rate.

Andrea

It was a Friday and it was the 13th of October.

Sonia

I had come on a late shift and I remember the postnatal ward I was on and the postnatal sister.

Lesley

It was a Friday evening and I was going away the next day.

Ann

I had just returned from maternity leave . . . I was on night duty.

Becky

The triggers and associations that evoked the lasting memories of the midwives varied considerably. However, there is a consistency in their recall of the exact time and the room where the event took place that still served to remind those who continued to work in the same room.

I was working on labour ward and it was Monday evening and it was in room 1.

Claire

The ward she was on and the room . . . I can remember . . . I go into that room and it still reminds me.

Janet

I can still see the lady, the lady in the bed in room 4, she was very thin and she was nearly term and I could see her sat on the bed crying . . . yes, yes I can now see her sat on the bed in the room . . . (long pause) *in room 4.*

Lesley

They were Alexandra wards and I can recall the exact bed she was in . . . my memories are so clear.

Sally

It may be argued that such associations serve only to maintain the midwives' ability to consciously retain these memories. However, in doing so they may allow a sad event to become an emotionally disabling experience. Janet and Lesley's recollections evoked strong feelings that suspended them in a frame of negativity that appeared to prohibit them from considering any positive angles to their experiences. The shedding of a tear, and a shake of the head confirmed their sadness.

I can see her five or six children around her . . . and she'd lost the baby . . . it was in the basket (tape turned off as midwife is crying). *I'll never ever forget that, and I've never ever cried as much.*

Janet

I could see her sat on the bed crying and her husband was crying . . . oh so sad, so sad! (Shakes her head slowly.)

Lesley

Janet and Lesley could have been enabled to identify the positive rather than the negative outcomes from witnessing such a scene, albeit a tragic one. It could be interpreted that these midwives were privileged to witness these events. For example, in the first instance, a nurturing mother was attempting to remove the taboo of death by encouraging her other children to acknowledge their stillborn sibling. The second instance showed a couple whose relationship was such that they were open to sharing with each other their feelings around the loss of their baby. Such positive aspects of bereavement are noteworthy for the midwife, who may be able to use this experience to help other bereaved parents. They are certainly worthy of positive feedback to the parents concerned and can thus be a comfort to all involved.

Positive and negative memories are stored within our minds, and mementos that we choose to keep can activate those memories whenever they are viewed. There are proud displays of 'thank you' cards in every maternity unit. They are a very public display of successful pregnancy outcomes and praise for those members of staff involved in each event. Mementos that midwives give to mothers of stillborn babies (locks of hair and footprints) are given in the hope that they will help the mother reconcile her ideas about what might have been with reality (Dickenson, Johnson and Katz 2000). Keeping cards from these bereaved parents was clearly important to the midwives and served either as personal tributes for care given or to remind the midwives of their own professional history of loss (Corr, Nabe and Corr 1997). They remained as evidence of meaningful events, carefully preserved, safely hidden, and allowed by their recipients to surface periodically to trigger memories and maintain ties. Lesley avoided eye contact as if she was too sad or embarrassed to confirm the importance of certain cards.

I keep the cards sent to me by mothers who have had a stillbirth . . . (looks down on to her lap). *They are meaningful to me . . . more so than the rest.*

Lesley

I keep all these letters sent to me from them, they are very precious.

Linda

As well as triggering memories, some midwives had used the comments on these cards as feedback on their practice, which could guide them in similar situations.

I can look back on them cards and see what I have done to help.

Becky

It is interesting you keep the cards from those who have stillbirths and that you see that as more important than those who have had live births . . . they say that I made it so much easier for them, and they make comments on the way I dressed and washed the baby.

Kathryn

Some stillbirths were more meaningful to the midwives than others and this supports Cutler's (1998) finding when studying nurses and their reaction to patient deaths. The midwives linked some of these events with their own impending or newly acquired status of motherhood.

The woman was 37 weeks and I was 35 weeks . . . I was going on annual leave and only five weeks to go.

Ann

I was myself expecting a child . . . and that would tell you that it is nearly 30 years ago. It's funny the things that you can remember and I can remember just what she looked like.

Sally

My own son was only six months old, I had just myself completed maternity leave . . . that's why I remember . . . I was a mum (points a finger into her chest and smiles broadly).

Becky

I was heavily pregnant at the time myself, I kept thinking 'what if? what if?'

Sonia

This experience was very personal to Sonia, raising the fear that she too could have a stillborn child.

Sonia and Lesley's accounts are linked together, in that they identified with mothers of stillborn babies who were themselves midwives. Thus their experiences informed them that a midwife could have a stillborn baby herself. The first three pregnancy losses that Lesley encountered were all delivered of midwives. Similarly, for Sonia, a colleague having a stillbirth became an important marker in her career.

I suppose I can't really remember much as a student, but later in my career I admitted a lady who was actually a colleague . . . that is my first clear memory . . . I had worked with her.

Sonia

My first experience is so important to me . . . we actually had three midwives having stillbirths or late miscarriages in the space of two weeks . . . I never got to see any neonatal or paediatric deaths . . . seeing those babies terrified me . . . It's the taboo of the subject of death . . . I was petrified (takes a big breath and puts her hands to her chest) *. . . I had been a midwife 3 years before I first got involved.*

Lesley

Lesley used the word 'petrified' adding a tone of voice that was loud and strong, and she sought to convey her shock by placing her hand over her heart, a movement of the hands that is held to convey a deeply felt emotion or belief.

Two midwives compared their experience of stillbirths to a previous threatening situation, or an episode of acute physical pain. These accounts highlight how one negative experience can fuse into another and create a meaningful event (Figley, Bride and Mazza 1997; Staudacher 1987). Becky compared two emotional experiences: a road traffic accident and a stillbirth. Vigorous shaking of the head and rapid speech is called 'self-synchrony', a process whereby the body of the individual is seen to move in time to the rate of their speech (Bull 2001). Self-synchrony is seen to accompany emphatic words that are used to convey deeply felt emotions and vocal stress. Janet's facial changes clearly showed that for her there was comparability between a physical injury and the memory of a mother who had a stillbirth – both experiences caused her pain.

> *This blackness exists* (puts both her hands into the air) *wherever you are . . . the blackness is still there. It was a horrible, horrible situation, for anybody* (speaking quickly, shakes her head violently) *to be in, it's like being in a road traffic accident all over again . . . I was so upset and shocked!*
>
> Becky

> *I know it sounds silly but I trapped my thumb on the bed* (wincing repeatedly) *and I lost my nail and it's grown back now but for weeks and weeks I used to look at my sore thumb and think of this lady . . . it was awful, it was awful.*
>
> Janet

Some of the midwives recounted events that challenged their own beliefs and values. Sally described her feelings when she experienced a clash between her beliefs, values and expectations and those of her client's partner. Judgements made by Sally were born out of feelings of sympathy and anger. The father of the stillborn baby is tainted as a 'Jack the lad' by Sally, for in her opinion he sought only to brag about his sexual conquests with a physically disabled young woman whose stillborn baby she sadly delivered. He simply 'used' her, in Sally's view. While midwives must not make public judgement on their clients or their families, irrespective of their personal beliefs and values (NMC 2008), midwives have their own social and family experiences and will inevitably hold their own views, which, though not displayed publicly, may surface in places of sanctuary such as a confidential interview situation. Sally's judgement of a father and the anger she felt was delivered swiftly and to the point. Her gaze was removed and her body stiffened, her anger was clearly visible. In seeking clarification of her non-verbal communication, Sally was probed further.

> Sally: *She suffered from . . . and not a very pretty girl, and without a terribly bubbly personality, that the chances are this was the only baby that she was going to have . . .* (long pause, looks across the room).

DK: *Looking now at your face and gestures, it looks like you are reliving it, you look very angry.*

Sally: *Yes. I am!* (Long pause.) . . . *I can remember so clearly, in my mind I am walking down that ward and I can remember the exact bed that she was in!*

Sally's feelings of unresolved anger prohibited her from finding resolution to an incident that was 20 years old.

A TERRIBLE WASTE OF LIFE

At some stage in their narrative almost all the midwives displayed a sense of dissonance between their experience of stillbirth and their professional expectations of birth and those of society in general. In contemporary Western societies, the advertised image of pregnancy and childbirth is portrayed as 'idyllic'. Few books or magazines display a baby, a toddler or their parents as anything but perfectly serene and happy. Boyle (1997) describes succinctly the magnitude of a baby's death:

> How hard it is to imagine an experience more at odds with this image of motherhood than the birth of a baby who has already died or who dies soon after birth.
>
> (Boyle 1997: 13)

The midwives constantly said 'what a waste' as they themselves struggled emotionally to come to terms with the tragic outcome. Their anger at this waste appeared to rage at times, and their confusion at the outcome was clearly evident.

> *I remember going down with the sister to see the baby . . . what a perfect baby, and I thought he needed to be shown off . . . for people to admire him. So we washed him and named him. I could genuinely say, 'he is beautiful isn't he' . . . what a waste!*
>
> Lesley

> *It was her first baby, she was 39 years old, so she was sort of at the end of not being able to do it again, wasted, wasted!* (Shakes her head and hangs it low.) *I thought it was all so really sad.*
>
> Claire

Portch (1995) explains that head movements can signal a great deal more than just yes or no, such movement can be a sign of inclusiveness. Also the feeling of sadness is depicted through low vocal tone and speech that is quiet and slow. This was seen in both Claire and Sally as they emphasised the word 'all' and their speech was at times barely audible.

I just thought it was such a waste, such a huge waste, and such a waste for this girl because she had gone away for the week to see relatives, and she had happened to go into labour . . . and it all went wrong! (Shakes her head.)

Sally

Just what a waste, what a waste, surely she had the right to blame . . . someone (speaking very quietly, head down).

Andrea

Kathryn's reflections took her to a position of understanding and being able to articulate and capture the essence of what makes a stillbirth unique.

I dealt with death as a staff nurse . . . looking after an adult who dies due to illness or an accident . . . but midwifery is unique: the mother is alive but giving birth to something which is dead (looks down to the floor, closes her eyes and shakes her head).

Kathryn

Kathryn shook her head and momentarily refused to engage with me (DK), effectively distanced herself. For a brief moment she appeared to revisit uncomfortable memories or she experienced a sense of insecurity around the profound statement she had just made: 'midwifery is unique: the mother is alive but giving birth to something which is dead'.

The midwives' accounts provided illuminating examples of how the stillbirths impacted on them, professionally, socially, psychologically and physically. The impact on the respondents varied and in some instances that experience, although many years ago, had left a lasting impression.

THE IMPACT ON THE MIDWIFE'S LIFE

Engel (1961) identifies how grief can be as psychologically traumatic as serious bodily injury, since grief can distort the physical as well as the psychological equilibrium of the individual to such an extent that healing in both the body and the mind are needed to realign the physical and psychological entity. Prior (2000), Corr, Nabe and Corr (1997) and Engel (1961) have shown that death can evoke many responses; one being that observers may perceive it as an irritant that impedes one's social activity. Weston, Martin and Anderson (1998) and McVicar (2003) agree that while healthcare professionals may be able to rationalise a death, or a distressing event, it is accepted that in some instances such events have a considerable impact on their social lives. This is demonstrated by Becky who displayed a degree of anger that lived on as feelings of nagging irritation regarding professional tragedies that had impacted on her private life. Susanna acknowledged a degree of psychological agitation that denied her sleep.

> *I kept thinking about this lady all through my holidays, and I thought, 'this holiday is spoilt', that sounds terribly selfish I know . . . doesn't it, but lots of things in my life have been . . . well my personal life . . . I've had this cloud over me about something that's happened at work.*
>
> Becky

> *I went home, and thought . . . couldn't sleep . . . rang up to see how she* (mother) *was, rang up again at past midnight.*
>
> Susanna

> *It only seems like yesterday . . . I can remember it so clearly and the impact it made on me . . . and my life then* (appears to catch her breath and takes several deep breaths).
>
> Andrea

The midwives had differing opinions as to whether their home was an acceptable place to discuss the ramifications of the tragic events to which they were party. Some midwives considered that home and family were their emotional safety net, while others considered it unfair to burden their loved ones with their professional distress. Within the narratives there is a strong sense of the midwives' need for help and protection for themselves and their families; the midwives' tone of voice altered as they chose to emphasise key words. One midwife conceded that husbands of midwives undergo experiential learning also: with the passage of time they learn that midwifery is not always a joyous profession; it can give their partners a 'bad time'.

> *To be honest I learned never talk to my mum or my sisters . . . I never talk about work at home . . . I keep it out! . . . Everyone is different but it's my way of coping really . . . I protect them and me!*
>
> Janet

> *You take it all home with you, yes, yes . . . you do it and it helps me. They – my family – help me.*
>
> Sonia

> *I went home very, very upset . . . didn't tell my husband because he is not a medical person and I've always thought, 'if I bring my problems home talking about it with him is not going to resolve it.'*
>
> Becky

> *Well, my husband obviously knew that I was upset, he knows I cannot discuss names or anything at home, but then he also gets upset about it . . . When you are so much later home at night, yes most husbands like him know you are having a bad time.*
>
> Andrea

Engel's (1961) theory that grief can result in psychological and physical disturbance and impair the body's equilibrium was demonstrated in several of the midwives' narratives. The words 'traumatic' or 'horrendous' appeared to be carefully chosen to describe their perceived bodily state at that time. The stillbirth is seen by some of the midwives as unacceptable, shocking and so mentally disturbing as to be experienced as harmful. The midwives' delivery of the words 'traumatic' and 'horrendous' was in a concise, precise and decisive manner, their vocal tones had a raw edge and their unyielding posture served to accentuate a further sense of their painful experiences. Becky, like so many of her colleagues, momentarily disengaged herself and all eye contact was lost. Lesley changed her body position; her posture was defensive and her hands clasped so tightly that they remained discoloured for some time afterwards.

> *When you have been giving them care and then this happens it is all so horrendous . . . you can be between a breakdown and normal . . . it can all tip you over* (closes her eyes and shakes her head).
>
> Becky

> *Horrendous just so . . . you are drained, you are drained.*
>
> Sally

> *I was so upset because of how I was feeling, yes it was all so traumatic . . . so traumatic* (sits straight in the chair, head held firmly, hands clasped tightly).
>
> Lesley

> *It can all be so traumatic.*
>
> Ann

Sophie's story is exceptional in that the mother had a normal, healthy, uncomplicated pregnancy and a home birth, the outcome of which was an immeasurable shock. She was the only respondent to experience stillbirth within the mother's own home.

> *However, at the point of delivery the baby failed to resuscitate and it just faded before our eyes. Nothing, just nothing . . . nothing made a difference. There was nothing known to me as to why this baby was not responding . . . it was gone, just gone there in front of our eyes . . . I was traumatised, traumatised considerably* (staring straight ahead, sits rigid in the chair).
>
> Sophie

Throughout almost all of Sophie's narration she made only occasional direct eye contact; she sat almost motionless. Occasional fleeting glimpses were made towards me (DK), as if to convince herself that I was still engaged with her, to confirm that I was listening. The extent to which the body is allowed to relax during interaction communicates a strong message, and in this case the message was interpreted as Sophie maintaining emotional control.

These midwives' stories support the findings of Figley, Bride and Mazza (1997), Corr, Nabe and Corr (1997) and Parkes (2006), who identify that sudden deaths, which occur without warning, require special attention and understanding. They advise caution as individuals can perceive these sudden events and react to them very differently from when death is anticipated. In addition, this study adds support to Boyle (1997) and Corr, Nabe and Corr (1997), who state that such events may be perceived as extremely traumatising for all participants, which here includes the midwife in attendance. These sudden and unexpected events could eclipse any other experience by the midwife of diagnosing or delivering a stillbirth or being party to that event. In Sophie's case there was no warning during labour that the baby would fail to breathe, as the heartbeat was audible as the head crowned. This community midwife had only a general practitioner (GP) present; she had no experienced paediatrician or midwives to support and assist her with technical resuscitation; only much later was she to learn that resuscitation could not have succeeded.

Sophie's repeated use of the word 'nothing' (*see* p. 27) paints a picture of a midwife making frantic but futile attempts, using all means within her power to resuscitate the baby. In this midwife's judgement, such an incident is the most shattering and in her words the most 'traumatising' of experiences imaginable. Figley, Bride and Mazza (1997) state that the trauma of witnessing a simultaneous death and birth can create a complexity of emotions that may confuse both the bereaved and their family, and one must be prepared to refer such individuals for specialist help. This knowledge, together with my personal experience of witnessing a death and a birth only hours apart and the profoundly painful experience of professional powerlessness (as when resuscitation efforts are unsuccessful), leads us to agree that particular support should be available for midwives in these situations.

Parkes (1996) postulates that there are clear links between grief and traumatic stress, and that what distinguishes the two is the character of 'the image' that pervades the memory of the death event or the lost individual. It is Parkes' (1996) hypothesis that the preservation of traumatic memories and images has meaning and is linked to loss of personal control. He sees these images as serving

> to represent a type of rehearsal. It is almost as if playing the memory tape again, one could change the way it will come out and regain control of a world that has slipped out of control.
>
> (52)

Sadly, the traumatic memories recounted by the midwives interviewed had not changed or been absorbed into the professional knowledge that they could use to help other clients. In some cases, these memories had stayed the same for many years. It seems that some of the midwives had experiences that closely resemble the post-traumatic stress disorder that can be experienced after birth (Reynolds 1997), as well as after bereavement, and is manifest with symptoms such as flashbacks and avoidance behaviour. If this is the case, skilled professional help would be needed to 'regain control' of this aspect of a midwife's professional world.

Andrea also used the word 'traumatised' to denote her intense feelings around aspects of a stillbirth and, as in her colleagues' narrations, there was unmistakeable non-verbal communication that emphasised the negativity of that experience. For a minute or two Andrea remained silent with no movement of her face or body, she appeared totally absorbed within herself then suddenly she started to weep.

> *Yes . . .* (a very long pause . . . looks out of the window) *yes because I mean if people have not had that experience, it is a horrible, just horrible experience* (tears roll down her cheeks, she closes her eyes and shakes her head), *but to be so traumatised by your first experience . . . so badly . . . is enough to make anyone want to leave the profession.*
>
> Andrea

Two of the twelve midwives thought that experiences around stillbirth could result in a midwife leaving the profession. Two community midwives acknowledged after their interview that they had sought redeployment due to their experience of a stillbirth. This study contains a small number of respondents and its outcomes cannot be generalised to the midwifery profession as a whole, or to the findings of Price and Murphy (1985). However, in their research report *Why Do Midwives Leave?*, Ball, Curtis and Kirkham (2002) suggest that difficult professional experiences, especially in the absence of colleague support, can cause midwives to leave.

COPING

When giving care around stillbirths, some of the midwives in this study experienced real tension between their wish to provide individualised care, informed choice and continuity of care, as identified in Department of Health policy documents (Department of Health 1993, 2004, 2007), and their need to set professional boundaries and to formulate a strategy that promotes self-care.

At the time of a stillbirth, midwives, like their clients, may be experiencing problems that are external to their professional lives, but which will impact upon their emotional response to the stillbirth. One example of this is infertility, for, like stillbirth, it does not exclude women who are midwives. Many midwives know of colleagues who have struggled to cope with their childlessness and show joy at the delivery of a child; others may choose not to discuss their own medical problems with their colleagues, thus hiding their personal anguish. Involuntary infertility produces feelings of loss (Mander 2006; Bewley 2010) and some midwives who have an infertility history must, on a daily basis, separate themselves from their own grief at being childless in order to work with pregnant or newly delivered mothers. One midwife in this study carried such a burden. These midwives may find, as nurses and doctors do, that their own grief may go unrecognised if they are unable or unwilling to communicate their feelings or if they belong to a group who may not understand the loss (Parkes 1996; Lamers 1997; Doka 2001; Wright 1998).

Some of the midwives who described a stillbirth that was meaningful for them felt they had little option but to encapsulate their own negative feelings for a variety of reasons.

To experience sympathetic connection to mothers who have miscarried or have had a stillbirth was deemed acceptable in Janet's opinion. However, she also felt that empathic connections between a midwife and her client must have boundaries, as they cannot be allowed to encroach upon her private life. Janet operated in a damage limitation mode; her boundaries were clearly defined, and were coupled with the fiercely defiant attitude that such events, painful as they are, must be contained.

> *I never . . . talk to my mother or sister or anyone about my professional losses. No, not even my husband. I just try and keep it all to myself . . . I try to protect them and me from hurting . . . It took me a long time to work out why I did that . . . but now I know it's about protecting my family.*
>
> Janet

Sally and Sonia reflected on their experiences and identified the reason for their self-induced isolation as being, in the main, a defensive coping strategy. Their body language and their spoken words were congruent. Sally confirmed that in the past there was nowhere for her to go to express her feelings. She inferred that historically midwifery supervision did not consider the emotional plight of midwives dealing with stillbirths. In Sally's opinion, supervision was improving in this respect but she did not elaborate on her belief, and in hindsight perhaps I could have probed further as to how a midwifery supervisor could adequately support a midwife in such difficult circumstances.

> *On reflection I have done that to myself, yes on reflection I have isolated myself . . . defensive . . . I have been defensive* (nods her head several times).
>
> Sonia

> *I never trusted again . . . for I spent 12 hours with a woman saying 'sorry' . . . there was nowhere to go with these feelings . . . resolve your own problems . . . supervision was not geared up for dealing with these things . . . it's better now . . . I now use reflection . . .* (nods and smiles). *Yes, now I explore but back then, I did not talk to anyone . . . we had nowhere to go with it.*
>
> Sally

In comprehending the enormity of an unexpected stillbirth, Sophie, like her colleagues, disclosed that she initially sought to isolate and protect herself from further emotional assault. This is seen in her diverting colleagues' phone calls, and in doing so denying them access to her private world. Some of her colleagues' motives she may have judged as lacking in sincerity. A simple shaking of her head enforces and replaces the word 'no'.

> *I had phone calls from colleagues wanting to know the ins and outs of what had happened. I plugged the answering machine in. I didn't want to re-live the story constantly*

(shakes her head slowly) *to every other colleague that wanted to know what was happening.*

Sophie

Seeking to isolate oneself at times of grief is a normal activity (Hockey 1986; Worden 2003; Parkes 1998), but one that supporters of individuals should approach in a cautiously sensitive manner, lest further emotional injury be sustained. These midwives had insight into their vulnerability to further emotional injury and sought to protect themselves.

Not all of the midwives chose isolation to help them to cope and some changed their tactics over time. It is assumed that their gregarious personalities enabled Claire and Sonia to break out of the perceived conspiracy of silence around the taboo of death and helped to shape their coping strategy for future stillbirths. Talking about stillbirths was considered by these midwives to be a 'healthy and positive option' and they appeared somewhat critical of other colleagues' attitudes and relationships. Claire's body language portrayed assertiveness and confidence that matched her tone of voice and the content of her narrative; while Sonia felt that she and her team colleagues had excellent working relationships that others, in her opinion, might lack.

I need to talk to people and to talk about this as well, but a lot of the midwives when we are talking amongst ourselves say 'you cannot inflict sorrow on other people' . . . I think they feel that sorrow is for them to hang on to within the hospital environment, and that when they leave, they've got to leave it behind; they aren't in the environment and so not in reality! (Firmly spoken, head held high, hands clasped on closed knees.)

Claire

Other teams have differing views . . . but we are six or seven in number, we have a very good working relationship . . . we talk together quite a lot and that helps us, we really do think that helps us all.

Sonia

A grieving mother sought and obtained continuing access to one midwife over a period of three months. The absence of any boundaries, relative to usual NHS practice, rebounded on this midwife, who was herself newly bereaved. Two important issues surface in this midwife's narrative. Firstly, midwives need knowledge of when to refer a client for specialist help, though this will vary with the context of midwifery practice (*see* Chapter 9 for contrasts with independent midwifery practice). Secondly, there is a need to acquire the skills to 'recycle' and learn from emotional distress (Deery and Kirkham 2007), in order that midwives may identify the reasons behind their actions and feelings around tragic events and learn from past experience.

I stayed with the woman the whole of the shift . . . She asked for my personal home phone number I gave her it . . . she phoned for three months. Her loss was hers and I had mine (the recent death of her own father), *but so many have said that they appreciate we suffer with them. There is a bond there, there is no two ways about it, but it mustn't encroach on being professional, but in the situation I have just described all of those boundaries were over-stepped . . . it's only now that I can see it* (nods her head and plays with her hands).

Andrea

Andrea confirmed what she said by nodding, but there was also a degree of agitation present as she fidgeted and played with her hands.

Worden (2003) cautions those involved with a client experiencing loss at a time when they themselves have endured a recent bereavement or significant loss. In situations such as these the worker may find it difficult, if not impossible, to function within that relationship until their own loss is resolved. This was my own experience, for I (DK) knew that until I had come to terms with the sudden death of my husband I could not continue with this study. I withdrew from it for over a year, not only for the reason of not wishing to introduce bias into the study, but out of a need to prioritise self-care.

Andrea's ability to reflect brought her to the conclusion that she must set boundaries and operate within a self-care framework should she find herself in a similar situation. Andrea acknowledged that she had learned from the experience, albeit the hard way. Wakefield (2000) identifies that some healthcare professionals become surrogate relatives following the death of a patient, as they are unable to step back from the caring interface. This idea is seen in several of the respondents' narratives.

I could have been more supportive by keeping a distance . . . I felt it was me, and only me, that could take that burden on for her. I learnt my hard lesson, that shouldn't be the case really. I have learnt that I must cope with things in a different way.

Andrea

Experience informed one midwife that the use of visualisation, solitude, privacy and appropriate music was effective in helping her to cope with stressful situations. Kathryn's tone of voice and word emphasis implied that she was able to dismiss and disassociate herself from the stillborn baby and concentrate fully on the needs of the mother when she was in her presence. Her 'wail' came later in the privacy of her car.

I coped with it then as I cope with it now. I do not think about it as a baby (shakes her head), *I think about it as a dark, dark cavern . . . I just concentrate on the woman, you don't have a baby . . .* (heavy emphasis on the words) *. . . I get in my car and I put an appropriate song on and I have a good wail all the way home. I do loads of things like that by music.*

Kathryn

Several of the midwives confirmed, after their interview, that they had sought a consultation with their own GP. Sadly, they described giving other, physical reasons for requiring certified sick time rather than owning the psychological impact on themselves of the stillbirth. In reality, it may be seen that they continued to isolate their grief.

Conversing with colleagues prompted some degree of guided reflection for Sally, Ann and Andrea, and that in turn led them to recognise a growth in their personal strength. Lesley acknowledged her need to be more assertive and challenge the professional decisions of others.

> *Oh yes!* (Nods her head.) *it has also helped me* (very long pause looks up to the wall) *in a sense to think about it given the same situation again, I would . . .* (takes a deep breath) *refuse to leave her. So . . . it has made me stronger in that respect of handling complex issues and how best to deal with it.*
>
> Lesley

Lesley's non-verbal communication appeared congruent with her spoken words. She was seen to acknowledge her learning by nodding her head and by looking up at the ceiling. The long pause, deep intake of breath and forceful intonation reinforced that her learning was profound.

> *If the mother wants me to stay, I stay, if she can stand it, so can I . . . and I must see this through too . . . I do it for a lot of reasons, out of my experience and through reflection.*
>
> Ann

> *I have learned that I must cope with things differently, set boundaries if it happens to me again and in similar circumstances.*
>
> Andrea

The contrast in the lessons learned by Ann, Andrea and Lesley is noteworthy and reflects their different situations.

Sally created humour in the situation when describing her practice of reflection, which I (DK), as a lecturer, would describe in more theoretical terms, but she confirmed that we both understood what she was trying to express.

> *I concentrate when I am doing something, I am constantly asking myself why am I doing something . . . do I really need to do this . . . I don't know if it is a good description really, it is difficult to explain how it underpins my practice now* (laughs and points finger) *– you've got a posh word for it.*
>
> Sally

> *Through experience I now concentrate on the needs of the father as well as the woman, and try and give the best . . . the best care that I can.*
>
> Kathryn

Kathryn admits that her experiences around stillbirth have generated positive outcomes. Through reflection on past tragedies she has gained professional insight into the needs of fathers as well as mothers, learning that has impacted on her midwifery practice.

Thus, the midwives, on occasion, used reflection to realign their own psychological positions and regain personal control. Lessons were learned and stored for future reference, and the need to formulate coping strategies was seen within some of the narratives. Those coping strategies can come into play before the actual delivery of the stillbirth when the midwife first becomes aware that all is not well with the pregnancy.

CHAPTER 4

The silent womb: perceptions of death and midwives' responses

The pregnant womb is anything but a silent place: the heartbeat of the developing baby, pulsation of the umbilical cord, maternal pulse and the sound of the perfusion of blood at the placental site can all be heard by ultrasound early in the pregnancy. These pictures and sounds, coupled with the activity becoming stronger and visibly definable as the weeks progress, serve to reinforce to the mother and her midwife that the womb is cradling a rapidly developing and highly active new life.

A midwife's range of knowledge and skills must include the ability not only to monitor growth, but also to diagnose deviations from the normal advancement of the pregnancy, including the possibility of an intrauterine death. The midwife is often the first clinician to raise concerns about the pregnancy and often the first person that the mother alerts to her fears. Following examination of the woman, if suspicions of intrauterine death or fetal compromise are present the midwife will seek urgent referral. It follows, therefore, that the majority of mothers whose infants are going to be stillborn will know before the birth, as will their midwives. This awareness means that the midwife is required to support a woman who may have known for days that she is to give birth to a stillborn child. This time lag between diagnosis and delivery can enable the woman, her family and the midwife to begin to adjust to the outcome of this pregnancy. In accepting the death of the baby, one can expect strong emotions to surface in the mother and, depending on the circumstances, in the midwife also.

The bereavement studies of Parkes (1996, 2002, 2006), Doka (2001) and Figley, Bride and Mazza (1997) highlight the impact of sudden loss on individuals, depicting the intensity of the anguish and distress felt by the survivors. They are all of the opinion that those with close ties to the individual, even if they are not relatives, could be affected by that loss. There is clear emphasis in the literature that the grief of those individuals may not be as intense or prolonged as for a family member, but it can leave them visibly shaken and with feelings ranging from profound sadness to shock and disbelief. Our study illuminated not only negative feelings experienced by these midwives as they undertook the professional care of women with an intrauterine death, but also their ability to clearly articulate them.

The narrative accounts identified how the midwives experienced the diagnosing of 'a silent womb' and how that diagnosis affected their emotional and physical equilibrium.

THE WOMB WAS SILENT
No fetal heartbeat

The shock of finding a womb full of 'deathly' silence resulted in several midwives experiencing extremes of emotion, ranging from high anxiety, shock, numbness, disorientation and panic sensations, to physical symptoms of illness. These descriptions equate on all levels to those identified in the bereavement, grief and loss theories of Hockey (1986), Worden (2003), Speckard (1997) and Parkes (1998). Examples are presented of the midwives' abilities to graphically narrate the emotional as well as the physical disturbances they experienced, albeit for a short time, during the stillbirth event and immediately following. Most importantly, their non-verbal communications provide a sense of congruence as to the awfulness of the position in which these midwives found themselves.

The emotional shock of diagnosing or being present at a sudden death may render individuals present as either talkative and erratic or reticent and stupefied (Staudacher 1987; Saunders and Valente 1994; Speckard 1997; Figley, Bride and Mazza 1997). In this study, several midwives felt stupefied; unable to justifiably express their feelings, they suppressed them. The midwives knew that they must always act with the utmost professional decorum as they awaited confirmation of their findings.

In these following five extracts there are clear similarities. The respondents' body language and voice intonations further emphasised the emotions they experienced at that time. The hand gestures of several respondents mimicked a heartbeat as they thumped on their own chests.

> *I just thought, 'I am petrified'* (takes a deep breath and puts her hand to her chest) . . . *you know feelings come back* (takes a deep breath . . . pauses) . . . *it's not there! Often when mothers complain of a decrease in fetal movements you think about it, and it wasn't there, the FH (fetal heart rate) . . . I was devastated because I had diagnosed it.*
>
> Lesley

> *You can feel your heart start to pound* (hits her chest with her clenched fist; she is breathing irregularly and loudly) *and your heart starts to rise into your throat. You feel the worse, cos you know it's not there (the FH) . . . it was such a blur . . . such a shock . . .* (wipes her hand under her left eye, she is crying).
>
> Andrea

You start in a way to start to panic (thumps her chest with her clenched fist), *you don't want it to be that way, you want it to be picked up, you want it to be heard, but you know deep down that you are not going to . . . and I just did know and it was such a shock!*

Sonia

Oh! It's just your stomach literally turning and it comes into your mouth and you just feel literally sick . . . (places her hand over her lower abdomen) *and while you are searching for the heartbeat you start sweating . . . oh it is dreadful.*

Janet

You get that awful sinking feeling when you try to get the FH on the monitor and it's just not there . . . (places her hand midpoint on her chest) *. . . How am I going to tell her, how am I going to cope* (shakes her head hard) *. . . and I didn't cope . . .* (long pause) *. . . I cried with her.*

Linda

These five accounts illuminate the physical manifestations felt by the midwives at the time that they diagnosed the stillbirth. However, they do not suggest that feelings of physical and emotional disturbance continued for any length of time or not to an extent that hindered their professional functioning. This may be because they worked in hospital and did not know the mother before the sad incidents, therefore they were able, like nurses, to experience a short period of 'professional grief' (Saunders and Valente 1994; Doka 2001). A very different experience was described by one midwife in the study who recounted a stillbirth at home. She chose to give an account of how she felt in the days that followed the delivery of a totally unexpected stillbirth. Her physical and psychological disturbances remained for longer than was experienced by the hospital midwife respondents.

Over the Saturday, Sunday, Monday, Tuesday when I didn't know what had caused the death, I lost almost a stone in weight (starts to play with her hands on her lap). *I didn't eat, didn't drink, had diarrhoea and vomiting most of the time – I was distraught – emotionally and physically distressed . . . and that's why I didn't want to talk to people . . . I bought an answer machine and plugged it in.*

Sophie

This midwife suffered the loss of a baby that was solely in her care during the labour and whose family she had got to know during the pregnancy. She also suffered other losses as a result of this stillbirth. The flying squad was called and care of the mother was quickly taken away from the midwife, not to be given back. She was suspended from practice within 24 hours of the home birth. She therefore had to cope not only with the stillbirth at home, but also her suspension from practice that lasted until long after the coroner's case recorded that the baby had a condition that was incompatible with life. Her loss was not only to do with a stillbirth and the loss of her relationship with the family with whom she had shared the bereavement, but also the loss of support from colleagues, and her professional credibility was lost for a long time. In her account the feelings of overwhelming nausea, bowel irregularity, unrelenting agitation and insomnia that resulted in acute weight loss and imposed social isolation occurred when she was suspended from practice. Such a vivid description of physical and emotional disturbances resembles the signs of an acute illness, and demonstrates how grief and loss can manifest as illness (Engel 1961).

Midwives live and practise in a technical world; they give service to a society that has high expectations, and failure and death are often viewed as synonymous. Despite technical advances and the move towards evidence-based practice, one cannot control the outcome of every pregnancy. This is an awareness that grows through experience, for, as one becomes a senior midwife, those experiences deepen one's knowledge of midwifery, which in turn informs and shapes professional beliefs and values.

Many senior midwives had memories of cases where the fetal heart may have been consistently audible with no deviations in volume or regularity then, inexplicably, no heartbeat was heard or recorded by the monitor.

> *Suddenly at 2pm . . . this one was five years ago . . . there was no fetal heart rate . . . initially at the time it was a matter of sheer disbelief . . . sheer disbelief . . . (looks sideways, eyes flickering . . . very long pause) I just went towards her and put my arms completely round her.*
>
> Andrea

During such experiences, midwives have to prioritise their professional commitments and this may mean that their painful feelings go unacknowledged, which can be deeply distressing.

> *I thought, 'I'll get another tracing done', this was only 2 hours later . . . couldn't find the heart rate . . . I felt sick! . . . I am looking after all these other ladies and I am in charge of the ward and I just felt panic . . . (long pause) I am absolutely wanting to cry . . . no one came near me.*
>
> Becky

Becky's colleagues did not come forward to provide support or care for her and she said she could not ask for such support. This probably reflects the culture of the service within which she worked (Kirkham 1999). As a product of this culture, it may be that Becky's own self-image and her senior status served to isolate and preclude her from receiving or requesting any comfort. Her outward appearance probably concealed the internal turmoil she was enduring. Yet her colleagues would have had the same experience themselves, so should have been able to empathise in spite of having to assume a professional demeanour for clients.

Diminished fetal movements: 'if only'

Lack of fetal movements may be indicative of intrauterine hypoxia that may lead to death if no obstetric intervention is forthcoming. Expectant mothers are told by their midwives to appreciate the importance of noting the movements of their baby in the womb. Such teaching is given in the hope that mothers will alert their midwives to possible problems and, in the worst-case scenario, to a death.

In this category, Ann and Janet described their experience of a mother casually informing them of diminishing movements. This casual remark alerted them to the possibility that death may be imminent or present. No midwife can be held liable if a mother does not act on advice given; however, it is generally accepted that if a mother alerts her midwife early on to the reduction in activity, there is the opportunity for positive action to be taken. Perhaps then the outcome may be different and neither party would view themselves as victims of tragic circumstances.

Ann's account is particularly poignant; she faced conflict in that her professional knowledge informed her that all might not be well with her own sister's pregnancy. Ann never disclosed her relationship with this woman to her midwifery colleagues or to me until the end of the narrative. Ann was at that time only weeks away from giving birth to her own child. Her verbal and non-verbal communication was seen to be congruent, a loud verbal 'no' and violent head shaking gave evidence to her frustration at that time.

> *You always say, 'is the baby moving ok?' She said 'no'. I asked her when it had last moved and she said 'last night'. I said 'Oh!! Last night!!' . . . (a long pause) . . . the lady then said, . . . 'one of my other sisters told me babies don't move in labour.' I said 'would you like me to come out and see you?'*
>
> *I wanted to take her in but she said 'No . . . No' . . . she'd go in the morning. 'I'm ok!!' But . . . I did . . . I did . . . I had to persuade her to go in* (shakes her head violently).
>
> Ann

Ann was seen to act out, for a short time, that role in which she felt emotionally safe: being an authoritative midwife rather than a sister (Wakefield 2000). In accepting that, there was a suffused sense of 'if only' emerging strongly from Ann. A fleeting shaking of her head conveyed a mixture of anger and disbelief that a conversation between her two sisters would reveal such a tragedy.

Confirming the diagnosis

Practising midwifery on an antenatal assessment unit does not require a midwife to deliver a stillborn baby, but it is often the destination for a woman whose GP or community midwife has detected a reduction in movements, changes in heart rate or a possible intrauterine death. Midwives working on such units provided accounts of diagnosing intrauterine deaths that were different to those from midwives working in other situations. In accepting that they are not always the first to diagnose an intrauterine death, they are often the ones to confirm it by using the Doppler or ultrasound apparatus themselves or accompany the woman while confirmation is made. Midwives working in an antenatal assessment unit may or may not know women referred to them, and the time spent with these women, albeit fleeting becomes a memorable encounter.

> *I've looked after ladies who've come in with no movements and then gone on to have no heart . . . dreadful . . . it's just so dreadful . . . you wouldn't believe it.*

> *Another time a girl came in, well she came to our unit worrying about the baby's movements and I always said to her that the tracing was fine . . . but I'm sure this lady knew that something was going to happen to her baby and . . . she was right . . . even though she had a heartbeat tracing previously the baby did die . . . I learnt from that . . . you've got to listen to the mum. Listen to what she has to say . . . give them confidence to believe in themselves.*

> Janet

> *She had reduced fetal movements for a couple of days. They had done a tracing . . . nothing fantastic, so she went home . . . came back the next day . . . got the tracing running but when I went back it had gone . . . I thought 'oh God, if she had only not pushed to go home we could have done something.'*

> Becky

> *I was doing a spell on the unit . . . this lady came in and the tracing showed acute fetal distress. I called the registrar but by the time he got there it was gone! I felt sick.*

> Andrea

These accounts show that the absence of a heartbeat produces 'dreadful feelings' and 'it is hard to be a midwife in that situation'. However, Janet acknowledged that out of such dire situations she has gained positive professional learning: to listen to her clients' gut feelings no matter what the previous fetal heart tracing presents.

An account of a midwife working on an antenatal day unit is included that afforded a differing perspective, for it related to a midwife returning to practice. Seeking to return to midwifery practice after a variable length of absence can be an arduous task. Twenty years of academic experience providing an educational framework and support for these midwives informs me (DK) that, returning to practice is a highly stressful experience for the majority of returnees. The degree of stress is often related to the length of absence from the profession, and the degree of support they have both professionally and socially is a crucial element. Such personal knowledge is supported by research findings (RCM and RCN 2000; Kirkham and Morgan 2006). It is hoped that any returnee in the course of their first few weeks of practice will begin to have the range of experiences of normal midwifery that will allow their confidence to increase and reactivate their prior skills and knowledge, preferably of normal midwifery first. For this returnee it proved not to be the case and the shock of that encounter was emphasised in her tone of voice and the violent shaking of her head gave the awareness that she felt this should not be happening to her.

> *The very first morning I was on the antenatal day unit, the very first phone call from a community midwife . . . no heartbeat present or heard . . . I knew her!* (The client, a neighbour of hers.) *There was a big black cloud in that room . . . It was horrible in that room . . . the silence was deadly . . . I felt terrible, it was horrible. I really think it's the worst thing, I think it's horrible* (shakes her head violently) *. . . I felt absolutely dire . . . just dire!*
>
> Claire

On this returnee midwife's first day on an antenatal day unit, her very first response to the unit's telephone was to bring her into contact with a woman whom she knew socially. This account identifies that another midwife may have diagnosed the intrauterine death initially, in this case a community midwife, but in seeking the confirmation of that diagnosis there was an impact psychologically on a further midwife. It is noted that the word 'dire' was heavily emphasised, for this word also means 'harmful' (Oxford Dictionary 2003).

INTUITIVE KNOWING AND WARNING BELLS

Midwives often share stories of pregnancies when they experienced intuitive knowing in the absence of any obvious tangible evidence (Davis-Floyd and Arvidson 1997; Olafsdottir and Kirkham 2009). This feeling of knowing can have positive or negative connotations; some respondents made reference to a sensation of 'intuitive knowing' or 'gut feelings' or 'warning bells'. Intuition is defined in the Oxford Dictionary (2003) as 'immediate apprehension by the mind without reasoning; immediate apprehension by sense; immediate insight'. This may be a very rapid synthesis of a great deal of information without conscious awareness of that process (Davis-Floyd and Arvidson 1997). Intuitive knowing is briefly acknowledged and discussed by several bereavement theorists (Weston, Martin and Anderson 1998; Staudacher 1987). The midwives in this study related their experiences around professional decision-making and consequent activities in certain instances, but could give no rational professional explanation as to why they acted on those feelings. Such admissions resulted in a range of emotions, from lively bouts of black humour to visible distress at the accuracy of their knowing.

> *I had worked with her* (a pregnant colleague) *and I got this gut feeling when things aren't right. You are listening in and you know that it's (FH) there but you've just got to find it . . .* (very long pause) *but other times . . . you feel the worst, you know it's not there. I think it's not just stillbirths, I think it is related to a lot of other things.*
>
> Sonia

You've got a feeling yourself with ladies who come in . . . this lady knew something was going to happen to her baby, . . . she was right, I felt so guilty, that we'd done nothing to prevent this happening. Believe them, the women, and believe in your gut reaction and intuition.

Janet

Looking back I did feel at that time the heart was not there . . . I knew the signs were there . . . I knew the signs were there.

Ann

It is so hard, you look at them . . . the confirmation is there . . . you knew it . . . you don't know what to say, it is horrid.

Susanna

Well, I call it intuition, but if I was more educated, more . . . (pause) I would say, it was something to do with problem solving, things like that, I was drawing on past experience, maybe I am subconsciously . . . but maybe you academics would put a fancy tail on, do you know what I mean (laughs), gut feelings.

Becky

Such intuitive-knowing statements may be dismissed as a projection back in time of the initial shock and disorientation felt from the awareness of the death. Others may argue that scientific theory can never diminish those times in life when connectedness occurs on a personal, emotional level. Intuitive knowing may simply be the midwives' accumulation of experience and knowledge, which served to inform them subconsciously of the susceptibility of a fetus to an intrauterine death. Intuitive knowing may be highly educated knowing, as midwives are taught how to diagnose the signs of distress and how to decipher heart rate tracings, and aspects of this knowing can be synthesised at speed (Davis-Floyd and Arvidson 1997).

Glaser and Strauss (1968) identify the dying trajectory where the pre-death phase takes place over time. An anticipated death can be prepared for and when it does arrive, however overwhelmingly sad it may be, it is judged by bereavement theorists as being far less acutely traumatic than a death that is totally unexpected (Lindemann 1944; Parkes 1996). The theory of a death trajectory has transferability to midwifery practice, as somewhat similar patterns brought on by physiological changes can be graphed and developing hypoxia can be seen in tracings of the fetal heart rate. The activity of the fetus may alter, movement is often rapid and accompanied by an erratic and fluctuating heart rate; then, with increasing hypoxia, fetal activity rapidly diminishes and death ensues. In the majority of instances the obstetrician and the midwife will make a prompt diagnosis of the physiological changes and will act decisively and swiftly within that time lag, or 'plateau phase', with the aim of securing a live birth by a rapid delivery. During this time the midwife is seen to act out her part in a positive manner for, statistically, the chances of a positive outcome are high. The plateau phase is not an opportunity to discuss anticipated death, as in palliative care nursing; rather, in midwifery it is a signal for prompt action to grasp the opportunity to save a fetal life. So, while it may be part of the dying trajectory, it is usually a trigger for emergency action.

Sally described watching the cardiotocograph (CTG) tracing and realising that a fetal death was imminent; this created in her feelings of shock, bewilderment, dismay, disbelief and anger. Her non-verbal communications gave further evidence of anger at the event and demonstrated how a midwife can take on the emotions of a victim in a traumatic event. The contextual elements of accounts such as this are consistent with the theory of Figley, Bride and Mazza (1997) they describe three distinctive themes that are commonly addressed by victims of a tragedy. These elements are also seen to arise in studies that looked at the impact on nurses of a child's death (Rashotte, Fothergill-Bourbonnais and Chamberlain 1997): (i) responsibility for the event (ii) personal vulnerability and (iii) feelings concerning control and self-efficacy.

> *I was much younger then and perhaps I would not challenge so overtly, but they didn't do anything, things were going wrong. The FH was going down, down . . . in the end the FH just went and we lost that baby. We failed to act . . . We lost a baby there and I really don't know why* (hangs her head and then looks straight up; looks very dejected and sad) *and I still don't know why!* (Heavy emphasis on the last few words.)
>
> Sally

Midwives Andrea and Janet concurred with Sally in that they experienced feelings of horror and disbelief at witnessing a fetal death, although evidence later emerged that these intrauterine deaths were unavoidable. Within the context of the narratives, one can hear the themes of responsibility, culpability and vulnerability. Personal fragility around loss of self-control can also be identified.

> *I put the monitor back on, there was fetal distress . . . the doctor did not believe me . . . I kept arguing with* (name withheld) *I phoned the consultant to say there was variable deceleration . . . the FH was going down . . . when I went back the FH was gone . . . there was no fetal heart trace* (wipes her hand under her left eye) *so . . . I stayed on just desperately trying to find a fetal heart* (tape is stopped while respondent composes herself).
>
> Andrea

> *A diabetic lady . . . she was for induction that day . . . I did a tracing and it was fine and she went home and when she got back in the afternoon only a couple of hours later the baby had died . . . I remember feeling so guilty . . . and I still think about these cases, you just think about them . . . it probably would have happened anyway but you just think, 'if . . . if I had got there sooner.'*
>
> Janet

Feelings of guilt associated with a sudden death are often expressed in 'if only' statements (Worden 2003); these feelings may be exacerbated for midwives by their professional training and feeling that they should be able to prevent such disasters. In our society, blame is common in such circumstances and women seem very likely to take blame upon themselves (Orbach 1994). The respondents continually expressed feelings of responsibility and guilt that were intertwined with some of the stillbirth events they experienced (*see* Chapter 7).

These feeling were often manifest as physical sensations.

> *I couldn't find the heart rate . . . I felt sick! . . . I just felt panic . . .* (long pause) *I am absolutely wanting to cry.*
>
> Becky

> *I didn't eat, didn't drink – I was distraught – emotionally and physically distressed . . .*
>
> Sophie

> *[I]t was gone, I felt sick!*
>
> Andrea

Diagnosing an intrauterine death is not a common everyday activity for a midwife; therefore when it does happen it can register as a short, sharp, shock that leaves them initially bewildered and acutely anxious. However, for some midwives such an experience can have much deeper repercussions.

These admissions of negative and disturbing feelings around the time of the diagnosis of the intrauterine death are consistent with the literature on bereavement and loss, which describes how people and events surrounding the loss may elicit strong memories, images and associations (Parkes 1996; Figley, Bride and Mazza 1997; Dickenson, Johnson and Katz 2000). The narratives of the midwives contain extremely graphic descriptions of varying aspects of the stillbirth events that form unique and complex pictures. Some of these pictures had been hidden, for such memories served to emphasise that these experiences had frightened them and impacted on their professional and family lives.

Their perceived loss of personal and professional control was certainly an important variable in the midwives' labelling of some stillbirths as 'meaningful events', and could be of professional use in future situations of loss.

Death changes many things, and it changed how the midwives witnessed themselves in these rooms dealing with the events around these stillbirths, silently moving around but always seeming to function professionally. It also changed what they saw, heard and now felt with their hands.

I FELT DEATH WITH MY FINGERS: SPALDING'S SIGN

The midwife utilises her knowledge of midwifery, her eyes, ears and hands each time any physical examination of a mother is made. As well as hearing no fetal heartbeat and feeling no fetal movements, the physical changes of death can be felt by the midwife. The fetal posture takes on a crumpled shape due to lack of muscle tone and angulations of the fetal spine. The normally round and hard skull of the baby begins to change shape also: the tissues of the skull become softer and the skull bones become loose and overlapping at the sagittal, coronal and frontal sutures. This physiological alteration causes deep ridges to form in the skull. The descriptive term for this process is 'Spalding's sign' and it is evident around seven days following fetal death. Approximately 24 hours after death physical changes to the fetal skin commence, due to tissue maceration resulting from aseptic autolysis. The epidermal layer of the skin starts to peel, leaving the dermal layer in the first instance, deep red in colour with black discolouration round the edges of the epidermal separation.

The changes in the shape and consistency of the fetal head can be felt by midwives when undertaking a vaginal examination (VE) to monitor the progress of labour. The tension, acute levels of anxiety and apprehension experienced at that time are clearly evident in these midwives' accounts.

> *I find that I really have to steel myself to act professionally; yeah when it is really macerated* (screws up her face and mouths the word 'sorry'). *It makes me absolutely cringe . . . It had been dead for such a long while. There was clear Spalding's sign . . . I was thinking 'oh God how is it going to come out?' and I thought, 'would it smell?' It was revolting!* (Grimaces several times.)
>
> Kathryn

Kathryn's facial movements added further accent as to the degree of aversion she felt at that time.

> *The last lady that I had to deal with, that baby had been dead for a few days and . . . when you know that the baby is going to be macerated. You know that nobody wants to see to that!*
>
> Andrea

> *It was four days after diagnosis . . . I did a VE and stretched her cervix without breaking her waters, there was definitely Spalding's sign, so then . . .* (long pause) *I knew it was on its way . . . but now I knew I had to warn her what the baby might look like* (heavy emphasis on the word 'it').
>
> Ann

Ann does not use the term 'baby', she uses the phrase 'it was on its way'. It was as if 'it' (the stillborn baby) was something dark and sinister shortly to appear to both the mother and herself.

Not all of the stillborn infants were in poor physical condition at birth and those that appeared normal provided a very different but equally sobering memory of the 'image of death'. The midwives who recounted dealing with 'a fresh stillbirth' spoke not of revulsion at the sight of the baby, but of overwhelming sadness and occasionally subdued, controlled anger at the loss. The narratives also contain an unspoken sense of possible relief felt by the midwives that the babies did not have any visible genetic abnormalities that may denote consequences for further pregnancies. It is interesting and important to note that none of the stillborn infants in the respondents' narratives had major external abnormalities.

STILLBORN BUT NORMAL

The term 'a fresh stillbirth' describes a baby that has died within the womb very shortly before its birth. These babies have not yet undergone physical deterioration.

> *We had this other little girl she was an achondroplasiac* (had the condition of dwarfism) *and she came in with no FH and I sadly delivered her of a normal little boy . . . so sad.*
>
> Sally

> *To see an image of a baby . . . a fresh stillborn baby but oh so normal.*
>
> Janet

The midwives' narratives contain various descriptions of what the stillborn babies looked like and the images of them they retained. In these accounts the midwives are seen to make judgements about how the babies looked, based on previous experiences of viewing stillborn infants.

> *Her colour was pretty good really, she was not black. Her skin was peeling in parts; she had only just started to go off. She looked quite nice really.*
>
> Ann

> *Yes he looked fine, there was nothing visible, nothing obvious, 33 weeks and 3lbs 3 ounces . . . he had a lovely face* (speaks softly, smiles broadly, but still looks sad).
>
> Susanna

> *You are really upset, you just can't help it . . . Oh and especially when you see this really good-sized, normal baby* (speaks softly, shakes her head, tilts it and puts her right hand to the side of her face, slowly smiles but looks unhappy).
>
> Sonia

Susanna's and Sonia's vocal tones were quiet and they looked sad, even though they smiled. Sonia's hand gesture displayed the 'fed up' sign. Lesley recalled with a sense of relief that her first stillborn baby was 'normal' and, most importantly, she made a value judgement in that in her opinion the baby looked 'perfect'.

> *In every sense he was a normal baby but stillborn . . . he was, he really was perfect looking.*
>
> Lesley

Claire's account was very similar to Lesley's in that there was a strong sense of emotional relief that she viewed a normal but sadly stillborn baby. However, Claire was the only respondent to make the positive statement that, even though the baby was stillborn, she was privileged to be party to its birth.

> *In another case it was really sad; I said a little prayer. He just looked so perfect . . . so normal . . . I felt so honoured just to be able to do that* (looks down on her knees).
> Claire

Images of people and events are retained within the memory, but they can also be captured forever on photographic film. It is normal practice for midwives or health-care assistants to take Polaroid photographs of the stillborn baby as mementos for the parents. If the parents do not accept the photographs, they are filed away in the woman's obstetric notes in case they are requested later. In the 12 narratives, only one midwife (community-based) raised the issue of these photographic mementos of 'lost babies' impacting on her. Sonia's account is important, for the woman in her care had sadly lost three babies in rapid succession, two of which were delivered by Sonia. In acknowledging her own discomfort at seeing framed in the home the pictures of these normal but stillborn babies, Sonia rationalised and respected the woman's coping mechanisms. This midwife's distress was clearly apparent, with strong vocal intonations and the use of hand gestures as she struggled to express herself.

> Sonia: *The worst thing was that she came in again and lost that, she lost three!* (Holds up three fingers and looks near to tears; tape is stopped for several minutes while she regains composure.)
>
> DK: *Were you involved with the delivery of all three?*
>
> Sonia: *No, not this last one but the others yeah! You know she had these photos all over her walls* (points towards the wall and waves her hand). *The first one, then the second one and the third one, I think she is now trying adoption.*

This unusual situation encouraged me to delve deeper into this midwife's experience and in doing so I gained awareness of her knowledge of bereavement support.

> *Just so awful . . . just so awful . . . sheer shock; yes sheer shock . . .* (tape is turned off; starts to cry). *You are just not used to seeing this, you see but, this is the way that things are now, and you must encourage people to grieve and work through their own process, do what they want to do and how they want to do it.*
> Sonia

Repetitive use of words or the over-use of emotionally loaded description, as seen in Sonia's account, is often an indication of high anxiety or conflict (Minardi and Riley 1997). However, by reflecting on these tragedies, three positive lessons clearly emerged: firstly, Sonia recognised that grief is a process that one must work through; secondly, if the midwifery profession encourages the taking of photographs for the parents, how they use those photographs must not be questioned; thirdly, no two individuals will grieve in exactly the same way, but all will need support from their midwife.

The sight of a stillborn infant resulted in the midwives experiencing negative feelings. Those feelings became intensified when the midwife considered that the brief resting place of the stillborn infant was not acceptable.

A SILENT PARCEL: THE SLUICE IS NO PLACE FOR A BABY

In many maternity units there is a small room where the bodies of stillborn infants or late miscarriages will lie until they are taken to the mortuary, or the baby will be washed, dressed and placed in a cot in the same room as the mother, unless she wishes otherwise. However, in the past, some of the midwives in this study recalled stillborn babies awaiting attention in the labour suite, and in particular the sluice, until the midwife could undertake such final professional care. Other midwives recalled the body remaining there until the parents decided whether to view and hold their stillborn baby.

The sluice consists of hard, clean surfaces and is associated with cleaning away waste products and rubbish, not with items that should be treated with respect. The length of time that the babies stayed in the sluice was brief; nevertheless those images remain for some midwives and they harboured feelings ranging from high anxiety to sadness and deep disapproval. Similarities were found by Rashotte, Fothergill-Bourbonnais and Chamberlain (1997) in a study of neonatal intensive care nurses' reaction to leaving a baby or child in a cold mortuary.

> *I'll tell you what I really . . . really hate! I hate putting the babies in the first instance in the sluice; it is so undignified, so undignified. I try to put them straight into a cot. You have all these procedures to do* (struggles to speak), *I move them out of there!*
>
> Sonia

> *When I'm on my own and it's in the sluice I find it really hard to touch it, handle it, especially if it is macerated.*
>
> Kathryn

> *It was this awful guilt . . . and looking at this normal baby in the sluice the next morning it was just hell!*
>
> Becky

There may be differences of opinion as to the appropriate place for a stillborn baby and responses can become less sensitive following frequent exposure to such events. Susanna's suggestion of a place where babies would be treated with respect was impractical, but the comments from both a doctor and a midwifery colleague were insensitive in failing to acknowledge her motivation in wanting a better setting for these babies.

I remember saying, 'Can I take them (very premature twins) *to special care?' and he* (the doctor) *just said, 'no leave them here!' I . . . yes . . . I wanted them to go to special care, so that it looked like they were at peace. These babies ended up in the sluice, cos there was no other room* (starts to cry). *No facilities for them, so I was left . . . left to put them in a cot in the sluice. Then the night staff came on . . . I went into the sluice. One of the midwives said to me . . . 'So what are they doing in here? So, what am I supposed to do with them?'* (Tone of speech alters and there is an undertone of sarcasm) *. . . I just did not think the sluice was the right place* (smiles then looks down to her knees).

Susanna

The image of 'silent parcels' is linked to the notion that stillbirths have, over the years, been seen to equate to feelings of shame and failure.

I think in the past stillbirths were a shameful thing . . . because I have this image they were wrapped in newspaper, taken by the midwives and spirited away, but for babies it was, you see, like something shameful, it was like (shakes her head), *they were like thrown out with the rubbish.*

Kathryn

This description of stillborn babies wrapped in newspaper was for Sally synonymous with past failure and shame, added to which, she considered that she and other midwives colluded in the practice of 'spiriting' the stillborn babies away.

At that time we used to deliver stillborn babies and they used to just disappear from the sluice area. Do you remember, Doreen, when they just used to go away? . . . It was as though we had drawn a curtain and something had happened and umm . . . the child disappeared and [was] never mentioned again.

Sally

Several of the midwives actively sought out the means or spoke of a need to make sense of stillbirth events. In doing so they were not only influenced by the image of the stillborn baby or its grieving mother and father, but also by the behaviour of significant others. It is apparent that obtaining resolution to a tragic event may be significantly influenced by the behaviour of professional colleagues.

CHAPTER 5

A stillbirth was given to me today: professional pressures, conflict and perceived roles

Continuity of care is strongly emphasised in policy statements on maternity care (Department of Health 1993, 2004, 2007) and we know that continuing support in labour is appreciated by mothers (Hodnett *et al.* 2007). Such continuity is likely to be particularly important where stillbirth removes the primary reward of childbirth.

Many hospitals have policies that allow the known community midwife, requested by the mother, to deliver or remain with a labouring woman in hospital. Then, if the mother is well, arrangements are made for early transfer home. Postnatal care is then completed within the woman's home environment, usually by the same midwife or her colleague(s).

Where there are arrangements for a community midwife to attend a woman in labour, some will attend the delivery even if they are not officially on duty. In contrast, most women who come into Finehospital for their labour are attended by a previously unknown midwife. Once the delivery is complete and the mother's general condition stabilised, transfer home into the care of their community midwife will follow.

This chapter identifies the perceived pressures of caring for a woman with a stillbirth from the midwive's perspective, irrespective of her area of clinical practice.

Several factors influenced whether the midwives interviewed classified stillbirths as memorable, one of these being how the midwife came to be involved in the stillbirth and whether she considered that she had any influence on that decision. Some midwives bore the burden of providing professional care to a woman with a stillbirth on a more frequent basis than others. There appears to be scant recognition in existing midwifery literature that few individuals can deal with death or traumatic situations on a regular basis without carrying a heavy and often long-lasting psychological burden (Doka 2001; Saunders and Valente 1994).

Several respondents utilised experiential learning, the role models of colleagues and reflection to help them create a two-tier framework for professional practice: on one level developing their professional competency and on the other developing skill in self-care. This enabled them to improve both the care they gave and their own coping capacities.

Several midwives expressed their sincere appreciation of observing and listening to senior midwifery colleagues as they carried out the statutory midwifery care of the mother and her stillborn child. The actions and words used were considered and analysed and those perceived to be positive were remembered and became a point of reference for future stillbirths. In stark contrast, three midwives were seen to judge other midwifery colleagues and doctors. It was their opinion that the words and actions of those colleagues at that time added further negativity to an already sad situation. For these midwives, their response to their colleagues' behaviour, whether positive or negative, remained strong even though the events had occurred several years previously.

IT IS YOUR TURN NOW: LEFT TO GET ON WITH IT

The allocation of a midwife to a woman presenting with a known stillbirth should be one to which prior thought and consideration has been given, but this was not felt to be a consistent practice. Some respondents felt they were allocated such a mother because other staff did not wish to care for her.

> *Folks seemed to shy away from looking after them . . . and seemed to think, 'we don't know what to do with this, and we don't know what to do with that, so you do it'* (points her finger at her chest).
>
> Linda

> *You're just left to get on with it . . . yes get on with it and manage; you have not got choices, I am so frightened of saying the wrong things.*
>
> Janet

Kathryn's statement said one thing but her voice was used to emphasise a hidden meaning and other agendas that she considered to operate in her clinical area: the power that certain colleagues had to influence another individual's 'luck of the draw'.

> *Sometimes it's just the luck of the draw . . . but then it just depends on who is on that day as to who gets to be lucky* ('lucky' said in sarcastic tone with big smile).
>
> Kathryn

Some of the respondents noted that, when they were allocated to care for and deliver a woman of her stillborn infant, there were marked or subtle changes in the demeanour of colleagues that were alien to the normal comradely atmosphere on the delivery suite. My own experience (DK) of losing my husband and gaining a grandchild almost simultaneously informed my daughter and myself that this is a correct observation. We both commented on how the demeanour of some of the midwives and doctors changed immediately when they became aware of the sad facts surrounding our loss.

Some midwives anticipated and understood why they witnessed these changes in their colleague's attitudes and even sought to justify their actions. There was clear evidence of a professional understanding that caring for a woman with an intrauterine death was difficult, but the perceived degree of difficulty varied. These three midwives use the words, 'desperate', 'difficult' and 'horrendous' to convey what it is sometimes like for them to care for these unfortunate women.

> *I was trying to care for a woman in a desperate situation because, you know Doreen, when you are looking after a woman with a dead baby it is always a desperate situation. It is desperate for the mother, and yes, so desperate for the midwife.*
>
> Sally

> *If I have been involved in their care it is horrendous . . . I cope better when I do not know them.*
>
> Becky

> *Sometimes it is more difficult than others, it is easier with one than another, it depends on a lot of things . . . when you have other ladies to care for too you have to keep putting on different faces . . . happy for one couple and reserved and quiet for these others, fearful of saying the wrong thing.*
>
> Lesley

Lesley identified that she had to keep changing her facial expression as she cared for more than one woman. Deeper emotional changes are also required. She conveyed a sense of emotional juggling and a fear of getting it wrong. This is a level of emotion work (Hunter and Deery 2009) that probably should not be expected of midwives caring for women in labour, despite shortage of staff, and which certainly reduces the midwifery support available to particularly vulnerable women.

Some respondents considered providing care to a mother with an impending stillbirth to be a heavy professional burden. The term 'heaped on' was voiced in one instance. The midwives expressed a tension between knowing and accepting that ethically they must give care to all pregnant women irrespective of outcome, and feeling that a 'no choice' allocation system was in operation. No one mentioned being asked how they felt about taking on this emotionally demanding work.

A factor that marks whether a stillbirth event was judged as memorable concerns whether these midwives were afforded adequate support professionally and emotionally during this difficult time. The identification of lack of colleague support during stressful times is seen as a major variable in McVicar's (2003) literature review on workplace stress in nursing. More generally, colleague support is a major factor in whether midwives stay in midwifery (Ball, Curtis and Kirkham 2002; Kirkham, Morgan and Davies 2006).

Some respondents thought that some colleagues avoided offering support to bereaved mothers or their carers because they sought to protect themselves against the negative emotions tragedies such as stillbirths generate. One can argue that such behaviour change by a midwife is neither professional nor ethical. However, a counter argument is that these midwives are human beings that have been ensnared into one of the cruellest life scenarios.

Lesley showed explicit and empathic understanding as to why some colleagues always find ways to avoid such circumstances. The origin of Lesley's non-judgemental attitude was revealed when she made the comment that, if she had the opportunity, she would also not willingly put herself forward to care for such a woman. However, there was some lack of congruence between her verbal and non-verbal communication. The hard emphasis on the words, 'don't' and 'they' and the slapping down of Lesley's hand may be seen as rebuking or punishing her colleagues for their selective involvement in such situations. Conversely, one may consider that she is punishing herself for becoming ensnared or berating herself for her own avoidance tactics in the past.

> It's my experience, like the other girls at the hospital, that it just felt like it was heaped on them. I often think it's about them protecting themselves . . . you have jobs that you don't want to get involved in . . . you keep well away, in case you get roped in sort of thing. People will stay clear and then they don't get caught in as the first or second midwife (slaps her hand on to her knee).

Lesley

These findings concur with those of Gardner (1999), who identified the avoidance activity of nurses around bereaved parents and the staff who were caring for them. In addition, Gardner emphasises that when death is expected, their colleagues' avoidance of healthcare professionals allocated to that patient is something that other patients and relatives see and understand. Gardener expands on this by adding that this could sometimes leave the patients, their relatives and staff with further compounded feelings of isolation and rejection. Ann met with resistance when trying to hand over the care of a woman with a probable stillbirth to other colleagues.

> I brought her into [the] labour ward from home knowing that there was probably no FH . . . she wasn't my own patient . . . No FH just the echo there, so I followed the midwife outside and I asked her to finish her obs (clinical observations) off for me, 'No,' she said, 'I'm not dealing with this one, you brought her in, not me' . . . I wondered if the woman had heard, thank God, she hadn't.

Ann

Similarly, Sonia and Claire's experiences served to inform them that colleagues often 'walk away' as they are operating in defensive mode. This empathic understanding was conveyed through a display of playful black humour. A colleague is seen to be baiting playfully with Sonia in a manner that implies Sonia 'call me in if you dare!'

> *The second midwife, she told me that she would come in if I needed her, she said to me but . . . 'if you don't want me in either that is just fine by me'* (she smiles and chuckles out loud).

> Sonia

> *Nobody wanted to go in, it was very much, 'Oh I hope I don't end up in there.' They said, 'oh alright then, I suppose if I have to'* (the midwife starts to laugh).

> Janet

Both Janet and Sonia may be judged as displaying inappropriate laughter within their narrative. Minardi and Riley (1997) explain that inappropriate laughter is often seen and heard when individuals feel insecure, have high anxiety levels or are experiencing emotional difficulty. Such laughter is often viewed as defensive communication, and a reactive response. Parkes (2002) stresses the importance of individuals having a secure base, within a family or a group, which allows freedom of speech and acknowledgement of personal feelings. Without a secure base, individuals will nearly always operate in a defensive mode (Minardi and Riley 1997).

Many factors limit the professional development of a midwife with regard to stillbirth. Lesley did not avoid stillbirths, yet the philosophy of continuity of carer did not provide her with the experience of caring for a woman with an intrauterine death for almost three years after she qualified. Lesley made an important personal judgement that, as time went by without this experience, her professional skills and capabilities could not develop.

> *It wasn't cos I had avoided it . . . and it wasn't people who avoided me looking after them. It was just how it happened . . . I was not on duty when people came in or anything . . . we try to maintain continuity and as such that makes it hard. You do not develop your skills you doubt your capabilities when you don't come up against it . . . it gets harder with time then.*

> Lesley

Midwives may avoid the care of women with stillbirths not because of previous negative experiences but from feelings of inadequacy and perceived lack of capabilities resulting from a lack of experience.

Lesley stated that a midwife may have dealt with death when practising previously as a nurse, but may not necessarily have seen a dead baby. Most student midwives now are not trained as nurses, so will lack even this professional experience. Similarly, when considering a midwife's length of service it cannot be assumed that certain experiences have occurred. Lesley did not say that any colleague had enquired about her experience. Ann felt this was important and one may surmise that she may ask leading questions of a junior colleague should they enter into a stillbirth scenario.

A newly qualified midwife, well now . . . could be one or two years before they have to look after or see an IUD (intrauterine death).

Ann

Attaining senior midwife status does not imply that experience has been gained in all aspects of the profession. Career pathways may change and result in some midwives developing specialist roles, while others may obtain a much wider breadth of experience. Qualified for over seven years, Janet had no experience of delivering a stillbirth; her work lay in the area of confirming intrauterine deaths. Nevertheless, her own experiences had impacted on her values and beliefs.

I've not actually delivered a stillborn baby, but I have looked after ladies who've come into the day unit with no fetal movements . . . I have come across a lot though . . . it has changed my outlook on how I look at a pregnancy.

Janet

One respondent identified lack of education or open professional debate about death as a reason why midwives become defensive. This fits with the findings of nursing studies (Lamers 1997; Wakefield 2000; Payne 2001), where appropriate education is seen as essential to help staff create strategies to cope with the intensity of emotions that can be felt in dealing with death and loss.

I feel that in midwifery we are not prepared for it, I know you can't always get training or experience in it but certainly don't think we are prepared for the physical emotion that we feel. I do think people walk away from it because it is their defence . . . just like having a bout of humour later on.

Andrea

The term 'physical emotion' is strong and apt. Andrea was aware that no midwife can be totally prepared for the emotional impact such tragedies may have on her. Yet if death were not such a taboo subject, some colleagues might not operate in a defensive and protective mode and they might stop 'passing the buck'.

PASSING THE BUCK

The difference between being left to get on with it because 'it's your turn now' and 'passing the buck' (shifting the responsibility on to someone else) was observed by several of midwives in the study, mainly those based in the community. Kathryn identified an important pattern of delegation of the care of mothers with intrauterine deaths.

Those who could not cope with the event, or did not want to cope with the event, give it away or pass it over to other people, the IUDs or stillbirths. I still think that happens today you know. When women come back to the community that is where I am based, you still see the same signatures on care plans for looking after those ladies.

Kathryn

It was suggested that these midwives were judged by their colleagues to be either better at coping with bereaved mothers, or 'easy prey', and therefore open to being passed the buck. This may be simply an avoidance strategy on the part of some midwives.

Conversely, some midwives were not encouraged to pass the buck when to do so might have been in their best interests. Where they lacked knowledge around boundary setting in the absence of appropriate support, midwives could naively choose to continue supporting these unfortunate women even though they might be at risk of emotional overload.

Linda described negative repercussions after her attendance at a series of working parties that discussed support for bereaved mothers and their families. She believed that some colleagues interpreted this as a loud signal of her willingness to provide the necessary support to those unfortunate women. These unfounded assumptions had, in essence, rebounded in such a way as to render this midwife a victim of her own interests. Her colleagues may have been naive rather than thoughtless in not considering the impact that continually passing the buck may have had on Linda. Conversely, they may have chosen to operate in self-care modes unchallenged.

> *I had been on a bereavement working party . . . after, I seemed to fall victim to looking after a lot of these ladies over the years while I worked on labour ward and later on community . . . yes, so whoever happened to be in charge . . . said to me, 'you go Linda and look after it.'*

Linda

Worden (2003) describes the importance of sharing the emotional burden with other professional colleagues when supporting the bereaved, and in doing so places great emphasis on the importance of considering the emotional health of carers. This was rarely the experience of the hospital midwives interviewed; they spoke of a culture of neglect in this regard.

The literature on bereavement shows that healthcare professionals should not leave parents to grieve alone (Too 1995). However, this should be balanced with appreciation of the emotional cost to the healthcare professional providing support. The midwifery literature does not stress the importance of self-care. This knowledge may be intuitive to some; to others it may only extend to avoiding emotionally demanding work. Skills in self-care, alongside increasing skills in client care, require education and nurturing in practice to avoid emotional burnout (Wright 1998; Worden 2003; Parkes 1996; Payne 2001).

In the accounts of two community midwives it is evident that their clients experienced a connection, or, as in one case, attachment, with the midwife that allowed meaningful interactions and deep, personal disclosure. Sadly, several respondents did not understand the need to set personal boundaries; the outcome was that their colleagues failed to look after them and they failed to look after themselves. In other words, they had no awareness of their support limitations and, as such, they become victims of the situation in which they found themselves embroiled (Worden 2003).

Linda made strong vocal emphasis on specific words in an attempt to convey how emotionally hard it could sometimes be when supporting a woman with an intrauterine death.

> *It had happened twice, she asked for me* (points finger at own chest), *wanted me cos I was her midwife . . . It was very, very hard . . .* (particularly long pause). *She had not got over a termination for Down's syndrome, and I was going back in after this perinatal death . . . I used to go in to her for hours!* (Shakes her head and starts to fidget.)
>
> Linda

Linda's verbal and non-verbal communication conveyed a mixture of agitation, exhaustion and sadness.

Andrea, like Linda, learned in retrospect that not creating boundaries when supporting a bereaved mother could impact on her in a negative way. There is almost a shift from being the known midwife to being a temporary surrogate family member (Wakefield 2000). There is clearly a link between the support available and the boundaries that midwives feel they need. For these midwives there was little or no support, so their resources were inevitably limited in the face of the mother's support needs (*see* Chapter 9 for contrasting data). Andrea found herself to be agitated and emotionally drained.

> Andrea: *She was phoning me to talk about the baby, what happened and what the baby looked like, she always talked like I was a very, very good friend . . . the phoning went on for three months!!*
>
> DK: *Do you regret giving her your phone number?*
>
> Andrea: *Yes, I do on reflection . . . now I do* (long pause) *. . . I realise now that I meant well . . . but it all went wrong* (shakes her head and smiles, looks agitated, plays with her wedding ring).
>
> *It was stressful, very stressful* (gives a half smile and looks down at her knees). *I would say, 'she needs to see me today', and they'd say, 'oh! Right then, you go and let her talk to you and we will do all your visits.' So, I did all of those visits on my own and my colleagues did the other visits for me . . . hard work. I thought 'oh my God what am I going to do?'*
>
> Sally

The textural and contextual composition of Sally's, Linda's and Andrea's accounts, coupled with their non-verbal communication, acknowledged that such sustained contact with one grieving woman was at considerable emotional cost to them. These midwives may have been feeling much more deeply than they had the ability to articulate (Figley, Bride and Mazza 1997).

> *I did all the visits, yes all the visits* (big sigh is heard) . . . *my colleagues just said . . . 'we will do the other visits . . . we will make it easier for you'.*

> Sally

Two interpretations of the actions of this midwife's colleagues arise. One being that the midwives simply opted out as a defence mechanism. The second, that Sally's colleagues may have genuinely but naively considered that their actions best served the client and their colleague by maintaining continuity of carer, and in doing so underestimated the emotional impact of such sustained support and commitment. In essence, they did not give her opportunity to pass the buck on to them (Worden 2003; Lamers 1997; Gardner 1999; Cutler 1998) or to discuss her experiences.

Similarities emerged in the account of a return-to-practice midwife who reflected on her experience of being placed in a care provision and support role, because she knew the parents socially. Accepting her colleagues' decision that perhaps she was the best-placed person to support the couple, she took on that role. It was this midwife's considered opinion that her colleagues had provided her with adequate personal support and consideration while she undertook this arduous task.

The managerial decision to use this returnee midwife to support the woman may be seen from two opposing angles. Firstly, that using that midwife to give care was utilising that known connection between these two individuals to permit the mother to have the best possible psychological support (Price and Murphy 1985). There is no sense in her account that this midwife was made or manipulated into taking on the care of the woman. However, this may be yet another case of passing the buck to this midwife irrespective of her status or level of competency at that time. It could be argued that the immediate needs of this returnee were to regain her skills and competencies in normal midwifery rather than support a mother in such a tragic circumstance. This midwife was, however, well supported.

> *I think it was just because she knew me, so we decided in the end that I would look after her as well . . . everybody was there to talk, it was really, they were brilliant the other staff . . . sister stopped coming in after a while she said 'I am here if you need me' . . . it was too hard for her.*

> Janet

There is an air of comradeship and no negative tone even when the midwife acknowledged that a senior colleague found the situation 'too hard'. Janet accepted that, for some individuals, irrespective of status, some things are just too painful to endure. Cutler (1998) described senior staff being able to have the assertiveness and seniority to opt out of some situations and Rashotte, Fothergill-Bourbonnais and Chamberlain (1997) highlight a similar pattern in observing that staff can and do develop control over certain aspects of their practice, a development that evolves over time due to the accumulation of experiences both good and bad, and with the attainment of seniority. In this study senior colleagues were seen to operate that choice, and in Janet's case appropriate support was offered by other staff.

Four of the midwives interviewed, while acknowledging the sadness and stress of a stillbirth, thought it was part of being a midwife and, for them, there could never be a conscious decision to pass the buck or opt out. This ethical decision was founded on their beliefs concerning their knowledge and relationship with self and with their clients. Their emphasis on their feelings of knowing the mother is interpreted as knowing her more than on a fleeting basis, having a degree of connection with her.

> *Do I ever think I am not going to deliver this baby?* (Long pause and looks up at the ceiling.) *No, no. Well because by doing that you are not facing up to things. If you know them as well it's very, very hard . . . gosh, I'm speaking for the team here and I shouldn't* (starts to laugh).
>
> Sonia

> *It takes great courage for these women, and I don't think I am being courageous in looking after them, you just do . . . get on with it, you know them.*
>
> Janet

> *No I always would look after them . . . It is just dependent on who gets it on the day . . . getting these cases is sometimes only luck of the draw you know* (smiles).
>
> Kathryn

The idea that approaching an anticipated stillbirth constructively rather than negatively could help to engender a positive birthing experience was found in Sophie's reflective narrative. This midwife was firmly of the opinion that, by removing the taboo around death and with adequate preparation for the event, delivering a stillborn baby could be a 'beautiful experience' for both the mother and the attending midwife. It is significant that she was heard to stress the word 'we'.

> *If we all had known what was going to happen we could have prepared for the delivery as a home confinement for the mother. This mother was scared of hospitals, that is why she wanted a home confinement . . . had we been prepared we could have had a beautiful delivery. I would have ensured that the mother and all the* (community) *midwives knew, we could all have had a lovely time.*
>
> Sophie

This is an example of considerable insight. The process of self-inquiry enabled this midwife to shift her state, albeit not totally, from being the victim of an unanticipated stillbirth at home, to one who is able to learn from her experience and re-establish professional and personal control.

Janet's narrative contains elements of reflection on practice and guided reflection though peer discourse. There is an acceptance that positive learning can be gained from all aspects of midwifery practice, including stillbirth.

> We support each other in our team to reflect on what has gone on, to reflect and look at ways. You see always, you must always try and make the best of things. We look at this and that and learn.
>
> Janet

This study has identified on several levels that through the utilisation of personal reflection some midwives were able to articulate the positive as well as negative learning that they encountered during a stillbirth.

LEARNING FROM ANOTHER MIDWIFE

For several midwives, significant experiential learning was gained by observing and analysing their colleagues' actions. Peers were judged on two important qualities: their professional image and their attitude displayed not only to the mother and her partner, but also to other colleagues at that time. In such observations the midwives were able to identify variants of positive as opposed to negative learning from the stillbirth. It is important to consider that this learning may have gone some way to precluding these midwives from experiencing the feelings of physical or emotional isolation other colleagues apparently endured.

Kathryn learned not to judge colleagues, but to be open to what she could learn from them and this provided an opportunity to formulate a client care and a self-care strategy.

> The midwife who had a bit of a reputation as a dragon (smiles broadly) *came in and took the skin sample for me, phew* (exhales loudly), *and she helped me to dress the baby and photograph it . . . she looked human . . . and I felt ok . . . I am coping with it, and I thought 'this is the way I am always going to do it'. It was a lot easier seeing the way she did it and looking at it and she talked to the baby saying 'you little thing, you have lovely hair'. It made it easier for me and I found that to be a good coping mechanism, she gave me insight.*
>
> Kathryn

Kathryn and her senior colleague connected with each other on a very human level and in doing so Kathryn's perception of her colleague positively changed and she herself became a more confident practitioner. Lesley had a similar learning experience.

> I have an emotional face; I know I react and show my emotions openly, I was wondering what this baby looked like. There is this disbelief, when people say 'does it look nice?' Are they just trying to get me in there! (Holds her hands tightly on her lap, displaying a sense of anxiety.) *Sister said, 'you come with me, we will go and see the baby together.' Yes oh! he was perfect . . .* (long pause) *it did make a difference*

with her being with me. It sort of eased the way, and I suppose the fact that she had actually been involved in the delivery helped me.

Lesley

Lesley felt initially that perhaps her colleagues wanted to professionally initiate her: 'are they just trying to get me in there?' It then became clear that this senior colleague understood her junior's fears and her leadership was a positive act that enabled Lesley to confront those fears.

The impact and value of senior midwives acknowledging the relationship between a client and their colleague and seeking ways of supporting both parties is clearly important. Janet acknowledged that colleagues, be they senior or not, must support each other for the stillbirth outcome to make a positive difference. Heavy emphasis on the word 'support' is interpreted as meaning this is crucial to Janet.

We support each other, you must at the time . . . we reflect on what's gone on, and look at ways, you see we must try and make a difference . . . learn from each other.

Janet

Claire (a return-to-practice midwife) had a positive image of her senior and super-visory colleague, which was later reaffirmed. However, she made unsubstantiated judgements that this midwife must have dealt with many intrauterine deaths; it is assumed that only substantial experience generates such empathic reactions as she witnessed on that occasion.

She (the client) *recognised me and walked straight over to me and put her arms around me and cried. I couldn't believe it was her. The sister who was working with me was just brilliant; she talked to her and me. I suppose she's there when a lot of IUDs are diagnosed . . . she was just brilliant* (laughs loudly). *She just stood and rubbed their backs and spoke really quietly and let them speak when they wanted to.*

Claire

It is acknowledged that all midwives have a duty of care to all pregnant and newly delivered mothers, whatever the circumstances. It is clear that personal and pro-fessional learning can take place even in tragic circumstances such as a stillbirth. However, this study has recognised that caring for a woman during or following a stillbirth can be an arduous task. The process by which the midwives were allocated to care for these unfortunate women and the level of support offered to the midwives emerged as two important issues when considering whether or not a stillbirth event was memorable. The decision as to which midwife would provide care to a woman with an intrauterine death did not always arise through professional negotiation. In addition, it would appear that these midwives were not always practising within a philosophical framework that identified and embraced the need to care for the carer.

THE STILLBIRTH DOCUMENTATION AND ASSOCIATED TASKS

Giving care in the NHS often requires detailed and lengthy documentation of events, medical decisions and interventions by all healthcare professionals. In the case of stillbirths, the documentation has increased considerably in recent years, following the creation of relevant guidelines and protocols. There must be accurate recording of events around the birth, completion of the statutory stillbirth notification and audit files. In addition, the pathology department often requires separate documentation. The gathering of information is supported by the obtaining of tissue samples from the stillborn baby that may aid scientific understanding of the pathology of intrauterine deaths. It is the midwife's responsibility to obtain those tissue samples from the stillborn baby in addition to preparing the baby for viewing by the parents, both of which are unenviable tasks.

The completion of stillbirth documentation seemed to weigh heavily on some of the midwives interviewed. They perceived this professional requirement as an additional and substantial burden at a time when, as the known midwife, they must seek to support and console the mother, partner and relatives. The account below succinctly describes the brisk professional activities of midwives after stillbirths and strikes us as a credible and truthful description. It enables the reader to gain some understanding of how the burden of the extensive stillbirth documentation may result in some midwives opting out if they are not supported by colleagues. Claire's body language, for example, underlined her frustration and anger and highlighted the enormity of the stillbirth documentation and her desire for support.

> *When there is a stillbirth the midwife who delivered the baby must check the placenta, examine the baby, wash the baby, take photographs, handprints, footprints; encourage the mother to see the baby and allow the parents to see the baby; then wash the mother, do her obs, see to the dad. At the same time, she has all the paperwork to do as well and I just think there should be two people assigned, and they should find somebody from somewhere!* (Clenched fists.)
>
> Claire

Over the last decade the stillbirth documentation has increased due to fear of litigation and the advancement of medical science. Knowledge of these reasons behind all the paperwork was seen to fuel tension and anxiety in several midwives and the consequences of documentary oversights and the outcomes of any omissions created professional fear and trepidation for some.

> *You see, the midwives are so frightened that if they miss something when either the mum has been discharged or the baby's body has gone, or a form has not been filled in right. Admin gets on their back . . . I think it is all quite fearful.*

> *It's always the same midwives who get to do it, deliver the mother and then has all this paperwork to do.*
>
> Ann

The paperwork, all that paperwork (shakes her head and raises her hands) *you are so busy trying to complete it all, afraid that you will miss something and get called in.*

Janet

Paperwork and the protocols are so difficult to follow. They are made as easy as they can, but the midwives are so frightened if they miss something (keeps nodding her head and smiles).

Kathryn

Kathryn showed empathy with her midwifery colleagues; there was congruence between her verbal and non-verbal communication as to the fear of missing out any aspect of the stillbirth documentation.

It's easier when you know you have someone in the background easing you through . . . helping you with all the paperwork.

Lesley

These narratives serve to highlight that failing to complete an aspect of the stillbirth documentation may have been due to stress and anxiety and is linked to the experience of loss and bereavement. Such sad omissions could result in intervention by a manager or supervisor for failing to complete statutory records. Sally displayed both frustration and anger at herself and her colleagues. She acknowledged that while stillbirths are less common than normal births, nevertheless, the paperwork must always be in the right place, and only attention to detail will protect her or any other midwife from managerial consequences.

It's not made easy and nobody seemed to understand on the shift because it is not something that you do every day, is it? So, I am saying, 'where is this' and 'where is that', it just made things horrible and prolonged (all spoken in a very angry tone of voice). *No, and I found that to be very annoying* (face changes, anger present) . . . *I missed out the stillbirth certificate!*

Sally

Sophie described being summoned by her senior midwifery managers, due to incomplete record keeping following a sudden and unexpected stillbirth at home. At that time she could only use the word 'they'; she and 'they' were then in a position of conflict.

The following day I was summoned to the office first thing . . . they . . . had dissected my notes (face changes and head is lifted up and held straight). *I had not countersigned my student's records of the labour and the care that day . . . I forgot them, I did not go back and countersign . . . I went home, sent home . . . so devastated . . . so devastated.*

Sophie

Unfortunately, this midwife, like her colleague, was so traumatised by the stillbirth that she omitted important documentary evidence. Sophie's and Sally's accounts identify an important professional issue: that support may be required for midwives in completing their records prior to them leaving the hospital.

Gardner (1999) identifies that following a stillbirth midwives endeavour to provide the mother with mementos and keepsakes. It is accepted that this activity is probably now universal; however, there is no mention in Gardner's study as to how the midwives experience collecting these mementos and completing the documentation. Likewise, there is little in the professional literature that highlights the difficulty as well as the importance of accurate record keeping at a time of high anxieties.

The stillbirth documentation procedure, as previously stated, requires the taking of tissue samples from the stillborn baby. This has been a midwifery professional requirement for many years. The midwife who delivers the baby normally undertakes this procedure. Only 2 of the 12 midwives spoke of obtaining skin samples from the stillborn baby and they found the task stressful. Sonia was seen to become distressed and agitated.

> *I just hated, I hated just hated it* (midwife starts to cry). *I am there apologising to this little baby . . . just apologising all the way through the thing to this little soul. 'I am sorry oh, love I am so very, very sorry' . . . I am trying to get this sample and it's so very, very difficult for me. No one would come and show me, that's . . . how difficult it is for us to do, I just could not go back and try again to do it* (shakes her head). *After some time I did . . . Oh God this really is it, enough is enough!* (Midwife is now visibly upset, puts a tissue to her eyes.)
>
> Sonia

Here is evidence from one individual that not only is the task of securing a tissue sample at times difficult to perform, it also may be emotionally painful to undertake or instruct someone else to do. Kathryn (quoted earlier in this chapter on p. 61) was very grateful for the help of a senior colleague with this task.

It is likely that the large amount of professional activity and record keeping that accompanies such tragic cases may lead some midwives to avoid caring for women with known intrauterine deaths. One cannot dismiss the genuine fear of the midwives of failing to complete all that is required of them in regard to the stillbirth documentation, as this may result in an official reprimand and a subsequent lowering of their self-esteem.

THE NEED FOR ACCEPTANCE AND SUPPORT FROM COLLEAGUES

Some midwives highlighted the importance of receiving support from colleagues who not only understood the needs of a grieving mother, but also helped fellow midwives to manage their own fears and anxiety. The importance of bereavement empathy amongst staff fits with the writings of Weston, Martin and Anderson (1998):

while every death is a unique event, to find another person who can feel the depth of the emotion of grief will reduce feelings of isolation.

Such a statement leads one towards the notion of professional bonding as presented in the accounts of three community midwives. These community midwives felt that a sense of professional bonding arises from understanding the experience of caring for mothers with intrauterine deaths. Canine (1996) proposes that grief is a social process and, as such, is best dealt with in a social setting where individuals can support and encourage each other to experience and share the expression of their emotion. This fits with the finding of this study that the midwives reported faring better with professional bereavement when they were able to discuss issues around death with supportive colleagues.

Sonia identified the nurturing that she was afforded from her community midwifery colleagues. Sonia also tried to bring the researcher into their frame of reference by implying that I (DK), too, as a midwife must understand their experience. Her laughter communicated the positive activity of her professional group.

> *I have to say, on reflection, I am much more supported by my team than I ever was before, yes, yes I really do. We are a small network, the fact there are so few of you, we all work the same and we all understand, It's like* (starts to laugh loudly), *it's like an old mothers' group . . . yes, you know what I mean* (points her finger at the interviewer and continues laughing).
>
> Sonia

It was Sophie's experience that some of her colleagues understood that she needed immediate encouragement and nurturing words following an unexpected stillbirth at home. Within the messages from the midwives to their colleague is an admission that many midwives in the course of their professional lives will have similar experiences, though they hope never to be in her position.

> *Several midwives were very good, they sent cards with things on, with little notes on saying 'There but for the grace of God go I' and little notes saying 'Sophie don't give in, you're ok, keep smiling, it will be ok don't worry.'*
>
> Sophie

The following quotations highlight an important reassurance that many individuals in healthcare seek to hear following a tragedy: that they are 'ok' both as a person and as a competent practitioner.

> *I think that sometimes you do need it; you do need support in the way of acknowledgement from them that you are doing a good job.*
>
> Lesley

> *I needed to know that I was ok.*
>
> Susanna

You just need to feel ok in yourself at times like these.

Linda

Only one midwife made direct reference to receiving positive support from doctors. In this instance, a senior midwife was referring to an unexpected stillbirth she delivered following which the fetal heart tracings were reviewed. The placing of her hand to her mouth indicates that her findings had placed her in a state of shock and surprise.

> *The registrar came in and you know, God love him, to give his due, you know we go on about medics being wise with hindsight. Well he said . . . 'Sister the tracing is fine, and there is nothing there to indicate this happening, you're ok' . . . he was kind . . .* (puts her hand to her mouth, and holds it there for several seconds) *. . . He could so easily have been clever with hindsight and said 'Oh, what about this then!' cos it just was not the textbook stuff.*

> *The consultant, God love him too . . . he came to me and said 'Sister this tracing done only two hours ago well . . . I can't believe it either' . . . he put his arm round my shoulder and smiled.*

Becky

In direct contrast, Ann described two diverse images of colleagues during one memorable event. As a community midwife, Ann diagnosed an intrauterine death and sought to admit the woman to hospital. The woman was as yet unaware of the tragedy that she faced and reluctantly attended hospital for a confirmatory scan. Ann attempted to hand over the care of the woman, who unbeknown to her colleagues was also her own sister, to another midwife.

> *I said 'I have just brought her in, you're the one on duty not me' . . . she said to me 'I am not dealing with this, you do it' and she just laughed, this midwife . . . the rest of the staff knew that there was an IUD in that room . . . they knew from the midwife who should have admitted her . . . but one of the others was kind; she showed real, real concern at me being pregnant as well, she needed to know that I was ok.*

Ann

Insensitive comments by healthcare workers at times of stress can have a real impact on colleagues as well as clients (Gardner 1999; Doka 2001; Payne 2001) and if not resolved can impact upon an individual's future ability to cope with stressful situations such as death (Payne 2001; McVicar 2003).

A degree of indecision remained within the experience of Becky as to whether the perceived image of her as the senior sister and a supervisor of midwives may have resulted in her being seen as coping, and therefore not requiring further support from her colleagues.

> *They were sort of being kind and saying, 'you're strong', but I wasn't strong really . . . I am shaking inside, I'm dithering and having to cope with this and all the other staff know something is wrong . . . I thought 'I'm the boss and I've got to carry on and sort it through . . . there is nobody to take over from me because . . . I'm the boss!'*
>
> Becky

It is arguable that this midwife's junior colleagues may have perceived her as a highly competent practitioner and only by confronting her and seeking to understand her true feelings, at that time or later, could they have encouraged any sense of professional vulnerability to surface. The concept of a professional mask hiding true feelings emerges in Lesley's narrative.

> *You get the most support from colleagues who are also friends . . . the seniors put up a front, they seem to be efficient and so you tended not to ask them anything . . . in case they dismiss your feelings.*
>
> Lesley

It is ironic that Lesley feared her feelings would be dismissed by midwives of the seniority of Becky who found her feelings went unacknowledged. This situation seemed to create a vicious circle of lack of support.

Confusion arose for almost all of the respondents as to how to cope with the emotions generated by stillbirths and whether or not they should display their own emotion at this time. The issue of 'shedding a tear' with parents or in private with colleagues, and how that is judged by colleagues, is discussed in Chapter 6. The impact on their professional image of showing emotion became a point of deep personal reflection, which was more so if emotional support for the midwife at the time of a stillbirth came from the grieving mother and father themselves.

RECEIVING AND ACCEPTING SUPPORT FROM PARENTS

Savage (1995) debates the nature of professional closeness or connection with patients and the perceived advantages and disadvantages, and points out that any therapeutic relationship is founded on partnership, reciprocity and a degree of intimacy, self-disclosure and mutual support. Weinberg (1995), Lamers (1997) and Rashotte, Fothergill-Bourbonnais and Chamberlain (1997) are all of the opinion that healthcare workers involved in the care and subsequent death of an individual must understand that the survivors of the dead person often have a need to thank people for the care given. There is emphasis on the important but largely unexplored concept of 'giving and receiving' from relatives. Lamers (1997) and Rashotte, Fothergill-Bourbonnais and Chamberlain (1997) postulate that patients' relatives need to give written or verbal gestures of appreciation of care given and received; not only does it help in the facilitation of their own grieving process, but also paves the way for care to be given again to them by those same healthcare professionals, should it be needed.

The ability to receive a personal expression of gratitude can, if allowed, act as a catalyst to social closure around a particular death (Weinberg 1995; Lamers 1997; Rashotte, Fothergill-Bourbonnais and Chamberlain 1997). In addition, the mutual exchange of gratitude allows the healthcare worker to assimilate their own personal thoughts and to realign any feelings of personal inadequacy; in doing so they are freed up to care for other individuals. This study identifies that the receiving of personal support by the midwife, on any level, from the parents of the stillborn child proved to be a very difficult and emotional gift to receive.

> *So, after this the woman said 'thank you'* (tape is stopped as midwife is crying) *. . . I thought 'how can she thank me when her babies are dead?' I don't know why I am crying now, cos there was nothing I could do. The emotion then and now is coming from the fact that the mother was supporting me when it should have been the other way round.*
>
> Susanna

The fact that the mother is bereaved but can still thank the midwife for her care creates difficult emotions if the midwife is blaming herself and seeking to make amends to the mother (Weinberg 1995). Susanna was seen and heard to emotionally acknowledge that there was nothing she could do, nothing that she could mend, so she could not reconcile the supportive attitude of the grieving mother with her distress over the loss. For several other respondents the receiving of empathic acknowledgement from the parents at such a difficult time also appeared difficult. Kathryn, Linda and Andrea struggled openly with the concept of parental appreciation.

> *Sometimes they . . . the parents say to me, 'that must be awful for you' and they pat my hand, and they think that you are human at the end of the day . . . I get upset thinking about it.*
>
> Kathryn

> *The poor mum kept saying to me 'this must be dreadful for you too, I am sorry'* (shakes her head).
>
> Linda

> *The mother said 'thank you' so many times to me, she said 'I know you suffer the loss with us' . . . it was awful she felt so guilty for being the cause of my sadness.*
>
> Andrea

It is noteworthy how closely Andrea associated sadness and guilt.

Lesley poignantly described how the husband of the woman she was caring for supported her as she was delivering the baby. Her sensitive account shows the response of the father and the guilt she experienced in receiving his support.

> *Tears were just running down my cheeks, and I can remember the man just coming up and wiping them away* (becomes very emotional and the tape is switched off). *. . . I had just delivered the head, not even the trunk, and there was he wiping my tears away . . . and I felt awful . . .* (long pause) *because I had taken him away from his wife. She needed him, and I suppose that made me feel worse.*
>
> Lesley

A visibly distraught Lesley was seen to relive her internal struggle that was brought about by the gestures of this father, and outwardly acknowledged her non-verbal display of her own neediness. A further account from this particular incident is presented as it illuminates how this particular father's human gesture to the midwife delivering his wife of their stillborn infant was an act of reciprocal caring. The mutual acknowledgement of emotional needs allowed both parties to find a degree of resolution that may have been denied without the opportunity to talk later.

> *We talked about it afterwards and he even laughed about it kind of thing, he said it made him feel better because at least he felt like he was doing something to help. Yes, his comments were that he felt he had done something to help me . . . and it had.*
>
> Lesley

Her narrative shows the emergence of a sense of connection on this occasion between the father of the stillborn baby and the midwife, even though a degree of 'gallows humour' is present. This particular father cared enough about her to acknowledge that she was not only a midwife caring for his wife, but a human being who found herself to be in a difficult circumstance. The reciprocity was a comfort to both.

Sonia stated that there comes a point of emotional saturation when midwives can no longer give emotionally and need reciprocal care to realign their emotional equilibrium (Spencer 1994); she also showed how difficult this can be to accept.

> *You just can't help but give to the point when . . . it is sometimes . . . where you have to receive . . . when it comes from parents it helps, it helps, yes. Because you do blame, you do blame yourself or you do blame the situation because of the circumstances. If it is in your nature to give, you do find it sometimes to be embarrassing to receive.*
>
> Sonia

Sonia's words show real insight; sadly, they also show ways of coping with grief through blame and giving without receiving support, which are not sustainable, and can result in compassion fatigue (Kaufman 1989; Wakefield 2000) and emotional burnout (Sandall 1997). The reciprocity, which is sustaining to all concerned, and which best develops where there is continuity of midwifery care (McCourt and Stevens 2009) did not seem to be compatible with the professional persona of these midwives. Their professional image could even render them unable to initiate the conversations that could help to facilitate a successful professional and personal closure to a stillbirth event.

Such tensions shed further light on why some midwives may not wish to care for women with stillbirths. These two themes of 'passing the buck' and 'it's your turn now' are linked to the enormity of the stillbirth documentation and the emotions involved. It may be suggested that such reluctant professional behaviour does not stem from a lack of professional caring. It is likely that some midwives operate avoidance strategies that stem from a desire to protect themselves emotionally due to previous negative experiences. It is only through hindsight that a midwife can reflect on the professional image that she portrayed at that time, and can challenge their own and others' words and actions. This is important in light of Lamers (1997) work, for he is of the opinion that without such a level of personal critique one is unable to recognise the emotional needs of others in similar situations.

These midwives collectively identified further elements around caring for the woman with a stillbirth that were problematic; these centre around the 'emotional labour' involved.

CHAPTER 6

Communicating with the mother: an emotional labour

'Emotional labour' is accepted to mean the management of personal emotions and the emotions of others. This concept has been explored in midwifery only recently (Hunter and Deery 2009) and is still not often acknowledged or examined in clinical practice. Nevertheless, it is an important and difficult issue in midwifery care around stillbirth, especially concerning communication in general and emotional expression in particular.

A normal labour is a time of great expectations as the arrival of the baby draws near and the midwife's work is focused on the relationship between the mother and the baby and ensuring optimum care for both of them. In the course of a normal labour, the midwife uses every opportunity to communicate and create a rapport with the mother and her partner. Midwives provide encouragement to the mother within a pervading atmosphere of anticipation, apprehension and intermittent joviality as they await the birth of her child. Once the child is born, the midwife stays with the new family, supporting breastfeeding as she completes her professional care and record keeping. In the first few hours following the birth the atmosphere in the room is seen to evolve from one of excitement into one of tranquillity as the presence and meaning of the new arrival is realised by the parents.

In stark contrast, death takes away the expectation of a new family member and, while there is still a labour, the birth may well be approached with dread. This changes the prevailing atmosphere totally and must influence the non-verbal interactions, conversational flow and the texture and context of all communication.

> *When you are looking after a woman in normal labour there is a lot of discussion about what is going on; you have little chit-chats about their expectations. The expectations have gone with a stillbirth; what is there to say?* (Shakes her head, shrugs her shoulders.)
>
> Lesley

Too (1995) proposes that when birth and death are fused together there is confusion of thoughts and feelings as well as a totally bewildering sense of unreality. Our experiences inform us of the truth and validity within this statement. In this study several of the midwives were seen to struggle through a minefield of complex emotions as they tried to establish communication with the woman awaiting the birth of her stillborn child and in the initial hours after the birth. Furthermore, this study fits with the work of Weinberg (1995) and Rashotte, Fothergill-Bourbonnais and Chamberlain (1997) in that, like nurses, some of the midwives' attitudes to trying to make things better hinge on acceptance: helping the parents as they move towards acceptance of the situation, and also the midwives' own abilities to accept that professionally they do what they can, and can do no more.

> *We try to make things better all the time; cups of tea, making relatives welcome, all the time just trying to make things better and you know that nothing ever can.*
>
> Janet

Nevertheless, the midwives did their best to support the parents through their tragic childbearing.

NO WORDS OF ENCOURAGEMENT TO GIVE

The midwives in this study attempted to perform their professional duties as they would in any normal birth situation, but they experienced feelings of alienation both professionally and personally. They conveyed a sense of functioning in a somewhat automatic state as they strove to maintain professional momentum. They described a cloud of pervading tension and anxiety. This pervading tension was underpinned by a fear that this woman's experience could be made worse by insensitive words or gestures. In direct response to that belief, every sentence that the midwife spoke was carefully constructed, for they feared that they might ignite the unstable atmosphere.

> *I try not to say anything that will upset them or make matters worse than they are . . . I try just to keep things moving along so to speak.*
>
> Kathryn

Communicating with the woman with an intrauterine death and her partner was considered difficult from many angles, but in particular in the giving of encouragement. Encouragement to help women cope with their labour is normally focused around doing their best for the baby and upon the positive end of the birth. However, when the woman is labouring with an intrauterine death, such encouraging stances, conveyed in verbal or non-verbal terms, are viewed by the midwives as essentially problematic. Encouragement carries with it an implicit sense of giving, and as such, these midwives concede that at the end of these labours they have nothing to give the women.

Communicating is difficult! How can you encourage them? . . . How can you remain positive for them? . . . there is no baby to take home.

Ann

Yes, you do have things to say but it is not the same; you can't have the same sort of conversation.

Becky

Lesley's account infers that there is more than one thing she cannot give to the mother. Her repetitive use of the words 'can't give' suggest that she could not give the parents a live child and there was little to give of her own self emotionally, for caring in these circumstances drained her emotional energy. Lesley's long pause, big intake of breath and negative head movements added congruence to her spoken words as she tried to convey that caring for a woman in such tragic circumstance was hard. The word 'hard' is seen to reverberate throughout this theme.

Hard so hard . . . (big breath and long pause). *I think it is mentally draining, trying to, no . . . no you can't give* (shakes her head), *you can't give . . . no you can't give . . . no words of encouragement, you are trying hard not to say something, anything inadvertently that will make it worse.*

Lesley

CONNECTION AND DISTANCE

The midwives were aware, not just of the lack of the normal emotions and communication experienced in labour, but also of the possibility of unwittingly conveying to the parents their own reluctance to be in this situation.

You try desperately to make contact through your body language, your demeanour. Language can constrain you and at the same time as I was trying to communicate . . . but also I desperately wanted to leave the room.

Sally

Connectedness was a very important issue in these midwives' experiences of stillbirth. The nursing literature also shows that knowing or not knowing the patient was seen to influence not only aspects of communication between the nurse and the dying individual, but also the coping framework of the nurse involved (Cutler 1998; Spencer 1994; Saunders and Valente 1994). This study shows that knowing an individual was seen to influence aspects of the midwife's ability to communicate effectively at that time of a stillbirth, and was also reported to affect her coping abilities.

You get to know the ladies; it is so hard, so hard.

Janet

It's much harder to cope when you know them.

Sonia

It is hard, so hard, when you know them . . . talking with them . . . Communication is difficult . . . I am sure I give the same care . . . But . . . I can cope much more objectively if I come to somebody who's having a stillbirth and I have not been involved in her care previously . . . but I know I give the same quality of care.

Becky

Becky sees knowing the woman as a challenge to her personal coping strategies since the meaning of the stillbirth is more personal when the family concerned are known. She balances the positive and negative aspects of the situation and concludes with a personal judgement that her quality of professional care-giving is not compromised by a lack of intimacy. This seems to provide her with solace and an ability to negate aspects of the event and render them less harmful to her; she does not explore the mother's viewpoint as to whether she would prefer a known midwife.

In direct contrast, Lesley suggested that knowing the woman eased the burden of communication; however, her subsequent statement showed that she still sought to leave the room.

I had at least met the couple before, so from a conversation point of view I felt more at ease . . . I said, 'I'll come in as and when you need me.'

Lesley

One is left to consider two reasons for her actions. It may be out of respect for the couple that she did not enter their proximity at a time when they were struggling to assimilate the enormity of the event. Or she may have been avoiding an emotionally challenging task requiring her to disguise her feelings of instability, inadequacy or reservation around instigating and maintaining acceptable levels of communication with the couple. Whatever the reason behind her actions, it appears that Lesley was trying to distance herself by completing her professional care and placing the responsibility on the couple to invite her back. She thus treated the couple as some midwives were reported to treat colleagues caring for a bereaved mother: keeping a distance that could make it difficult for the person on whom the onus is placed to call them.

Defey (1995) and Too (1995) suggest that some midwives may distance themselves from clients who ask searching questions around aspects of infant death and subsequent labour experience. Not all the midwives in our study reported operating in this manner. Though aware of her shortcoming and a long gap in her practice, a midwife undertaking a return-to-practice programme responded to what some may perceive as a daunting communication challenge. This midwife approached her task by utilising a hospital policy document creatively as a framework through which communication channels could operate. In essence, the policy became her guide and support so she could capitalise on the opportunity to fulfil both the woman's needs and her own. Claire's sadness for the woman was present in her eyes, head movement, and several times she took her gaze away.

> *I've been out of practice for 12 years . . . I just talked about the whole lot, just every-thing with them. There was a procedure, there was a sheet that you go through but it usually happens after the baby's born . . . I'd got all the information beforehand but it was just, it was the only thing she really wanted to talk about was what was going to happen next* (shakes her head slowly, takes her gaze away).
>
> Claire

Claire was the only respondent to describe the difficulty that midwives may face when seeking to communicate the reasoning behind obstetric protocols linked to intrauterine deaths. Often the woman and her partner express concern that such protocols, which advocate the induction of labour with a view to achieving a normal vaginal delivery of their stillborn child, are neither ethically nor morally acceptable. They desire only that their ordeal be brought to a swift conclusion by a caesarean section. This couple's ability to focus the attending midwife's conversation around one topic lasted for a long time. Claire's non-verbal communication of slapping her hands down on her knees suggested that whatever she said to the couple was not acceptable.

> *She was horrified* (puts her hand up in the air) *because, she was going to have to be induced and she had thought that she was just going to have a caesarean so she really didn't like that, so we had a long, long talk about why she should be induced* (slaps her hands down on her knees).
>
> Claire

The statistical likelihood of morbidity for the mother is reduced with the induction of labour and a subsequent normal vaginal delivery (Department of Health 1999, 2003). Accepting that such protocols are evidence-based, a glaring omission from these scientific statements emerges in the lack of due consideration for the psychological depth of fear, anxiety and even anger that such professed protocols may generate in a bereaved woman. Seeking to apply theory to practice is not always an easy task, and in these circumstances it is often the midwife who must convince the woman and her partner that, in the long term, this obstetric management protocol is in the best interests of the mother.

Claire's priorities were evident: to provide support, maintain communication and then provide the couple with evidence-based explanations and to corroborate these with her medical colleagues. It is the midwife's role to listen to the mother and facilitate information exchange, should it be required. Nevertheless, it is not easy to achieve this.

The studies of Too (1995) and Defey (1995) fail to examine how the midwifery philosophy of continuity of carer may be very hard for the midwife when caring for a woman with an intrauterine death. No mention is made of the fact that doctors, unlike midwives, are not required to be continuously present during the woman's labour and the subsequent delivery of her stillborn child, unless complications develop. Moreover, the midwife is required to provide professional care in an atmosphere that is likely to be sad, fearful or anxiety-laden and this is personally challenging over a prolonged period of time.

> *I spent the complete eight-hour shift with the couple; doing what I could . . . it was long and so hard.*
>
> Sonia

> *I was to look after this lady for the whole day; it seemed like an eternity . . . phew.*
>
> Caroline

> *I stayed with the woman for the whole of the time, yes all the time.*
>
> Janet

> *I stayed with the woman for the whole of the shift.*
>
> Andrea

Sally's repetitive use of the word 'exhausted' and the presence of long reflective pauses indicated congruence between her words and her non-verbal communication. Her lack of energy was felt as she attempted to convey the personal impact of managing some stillbirths.

> *It's an arduous shift sometimes, you are physically and psychologically exhausted, you are just . . .* (very long pause and eye contact removed) *totally exhausted . . .* (long pause again) *just exhausted. I had to deal with it for a full late shift and I went home absolutely physically exhausted and emotionally drained.*
>
> Sally

Midwives must communicate with and provide care to women from many differing ethnic backgrounds. The majority of the ethnic minority childbearing women in the localities of this study are second- and third-generation immigrants, but their common language may not necessarily be English, which creates problems in communication for midwives. In the current study, only three midwives made direct reference to ethnicity; within these three accounts, language barriers and suppositions concerning religion and philosophical beliefs inevitably influenced the midwife's verbal interaction with her client. These accounts contain evidence of how the midwife may reflect on her role and her ability to be the woman's advocate at a time of immeasurable stress. The midwives were still trying to be there for these unfortunate women.

> *I was working through a difficult situation, through a triangle, I could only communicate through her husband . . . You try desperately to make contact with your body*

language and your demeanour . . . trying to make the woman understand that you are there for her.

Sally

It is hard when there is a language problem. It was so hard just going through and explaining everything and that she did understand, and trying to clarify everything . . . Her husband had a tendency to take over and make decisions for her. I was trying not to be rude, but I kept on saying that I needed to know what her views are. By saying to him, 'I do appreciate how you feel but what about your wife.'

Lesley

Some of the Asian ladies will say to you, 'that is how it is' . . . they have a more philosophical sort of idea about it and sometimes they say, 'it was meant to be' . . . (puts both hands slightly in the air). But I don't know, I don't know what the answer is there . . . (long pause) no I don't know, but communication is sometimes a problem on both sides, and other times it is not.

Janet

Janet's account identifies a quandary around whether or not the perceived philosophical attitude to death in Asian women has its foundations in religious beliefs that allow the apparent unquestionable acceptance of the death of their baby. Laungani (1995) postulates that religious faith may offer some degree of consolation to both the mother and the healthcare professional, but highlights the need for healthcare workers to confirm that this is the case and not to presume it to be.

Some midwives, for complex and personal reasons, choose to remove themselves physically from the environment of the labouring woman or remove themselves psychologically by some form of robotic functioning. This professional activity Garratt (2010) describes using the psychological term 'dissociation': emotional withdrawal from a situation as a coping measure to diminish its traumatic impact on the self. They can be seen to be protecting themselves in a situation of powerlessness, which is the opposite of their normal daily professional activity.

Once the delivery is completed there is a change, from the numbness, almost silent and sometimes robotic functioning when waiting for the birth, to professional busyness after the stillbirth. This is partly because of the many tasks the midwife is then required to complete and partly because of a desire to ease the tension in the situation by whatever means she can, by trying to make a tragic situation slightly better.

TRYING TO MAKE IT BETTER: PRESENTING THE DEAD BABY

Most of the midwives interviewed acknowledged the feelings of anxiety and profound sadness that surrounded their final acts of care: those of weighing, washing and dressing the baby prior to viewing by the couple. This study supports the findings of Rashotte, Fothergill-Bourbonnais and Chamberlain (1997) in that neonatal and paediatric nurses equally found such activity distressing. These activities under normal situations are considered by midwives to be highly pleasurable, and this is coupled with an immense sense of satisfaction that all parties in the event have attained their individual goals. The way the midwife treats the dead baby may be seen as a ritualistic attempt to bring some semblance of normality into the event. Some of these accounts describe the midwives talking to the dead babies as they wash and dress them. The action is no different to that observed if the child was alive; the words similarly given, but with a tone that appears to be more anxiety laden. I (MK) have certainly done this, as a means of demonstrating to fearful parents that I see their baby as beautiful and acceptable, and hoping they may therefore feel they can look at and hold their baby. Such activity can be seen as a means by which, when faced with death, the bereaved individual will often aimlessly or ritualistically attempt to fill that void (Dickenson, Johnson and Katz 2000). Weinberg (1995) conceptualises that such activities are not merely professional actions but ones that are grounded in an individual's instinctive desire to balance the feelings of self-blame. Weinberg proposes that one's feelings of negativity can be invalidated by engaging in commendable actions, the offshoot being that such actions may enhance one's self-regard. The accounts now presented illuminate the activity of the midwives as they strove to fulfil their professional duties and to make the stillborn babies' appearance as aesthetically pleasing as possible.

> *Even the very, very little ones I try to make them look nice, dress them and things.*
>
> Susanna

> *I always make the comment about the hair like 'it's a little baldy' or 'it's got lots of hair' and I comment on the fingernails, I go 'oh oh! what lovely hands and fingers it has, just look at what your baby has got, look at that'.*
>
> Kathryn

> *Just simply talking and acknowledging his colour of hair what he had now and what he, the baby, would have probably have ended up like . . . She had dark . . . very dark hair and her husband was very blonde* (gives a half smile).
>
> Lesley

Weinberg (1995) stipulates that mourners who blame themselves often try the hardest to make some amends. Examples are present in the narratives of the midwives struggling to enthuse the mother and father into being part of the adulation of their stillborn infant. It is the textural content of their accounts that surfaces to emphasise the outpouring of emotional energy as they 'try to make it better' for the couples. The midwives' distress was clearly evident not only in their intonations in these narrative extracts, but also in their emotional outbursts.

> *You* (points finger at researcher), *many of us give 100% but you still can't make everything all right. So . . . you go on doing what you can, trying to make it better in whatever way you can for them, even doing little things for them. I was trying to take*

the pain and the burden away from her, which of course I couldn't do. I was trying to make it better for her (starts to cry).

Andrea

We did everything that we usually do with them. We kept the baby in the room, we didn't take it out to wash it (starts to cry . . . long pause). *We let her choose the clothes . . . but while the dad held the baby, the mother did not move to touch her at all* (tape is stopped; midwife is still crying).

Claire

Two concurrent accounts are presented from Sonia's narrative, which succinctly describe her feelings of sheer desperation as she sought to make things better. Feelings of negativity in this midwife are considered to stem from two sources: firstly, she considers that her professional actions are assaulting the stillborn baby, and secondly, her best efforts to render the infant more acceptable fail to impress the father of the baby and she felt criticised.

Sonia: *I tried to dress him* (struggles to speak) *and make him look presentable for his mum and dad you know, sometimes there is nothing much you can do to make it any better. Oh, well . . . I thought he looked really awful at first and we, I mean I took loads of photos and tried to make him better, to make him look nice. Then . . . but his dad said 'Please, can't you make him look any better?' Cos he had these marks now on his face.*

DK: *Was he macerated?*

Sonia: *Yes! . . . A little on one side and he had got quite a bit of vernix and I had to say, 'I will really do my best', but I knew that I couldn't make it better . . . couldn't make it better for them. I washed him oh so very carefully but you know, don't you, there are some things you cannot hide, and I know that they were a bit upset. I really tried my hardest* (starts to laugh and cry at the same time). *There was I talking away to him as I was doing it. Yes, yes* (crying a little at this point; takes a tissue but does not use it).

Negative feelings of failing deceased individuals or their survivors are recognised in individuals who are experiencing bereavement (Weston, Martin and Anderson 1998; Wakefield 2000). While, for close relatives of the deceased, these feelings may be more intense or prolonged, they are, nevertheless, emotions that are seen in the literature on the impact of patient deaths on nurses (Spencer 1994; Rashotte, Fothergill-Bourbonnais and Chamberlain 1997; Cutler 1998) and as such there is resonance in this study.

This study highlights the fact that, in the absence of any additional obstetric complication, it is the midwife and not the medical house officer or consultant obstetrician who will be required to deliver and handle the body of the macerated baby as they prepare it for parental viewing. It is accepted that such situations are not a daily occurrence in midwifery practice, but neither are they so rare as to be disregarded. We have no knowledge as to the extent to which midwives are given the opportunity to discuss how they may handle this professional requirement.

These accounts contain graphic descriptions of the experience of handling a stillborn baby whose skin was starting to macerate. Beneath these descriptions is a profusion of guilt that the midwives harboured against themselves for having feelings of repulsion towards the baby. Several of the midwives bravely admitted to the difficulty of attempting to camouflage those feelings of repulsion, even when they were earnestly trying to make the situation better for the parents. Their spoken words and non-verbal communication at all times were considered to be congruent.

> *It makes me absolutely cringe* (screws up her face). *It had been dead for such a long while. I thought 'God . . . how is it going to come out', and I thought it would smell and I would be retching. I must not let my face give myself away . . . I find that I really have to steel myself . . . That is hard but I do try my best and to get the baby to look as good as possible for the parents* (slaps her hands down hard on to her knees).
>
> Kathryn

Kathryn berated herself for acknowledging her personal feelings during the narration, slapped her own knees and felt it necessary to apologise for her words and insinuations.

> *Later we undressed the baby again to show the mother that her baby was not a monster, but the skin was starting to peel, the baby was macerated but not that bad . . . but still not nice, you know* (screws up the corners of her mouth).
>
> Sonia

> *The last lady that I had to deal with, that baby had been dead for a few days and, no, I mean . . . when you know that the baby is going to be macerated. You know, that nobody wants to see to that woman* (shakes her head and looks very sad). *Nobody wants to have to do things, everybody wants to run away from it . . . some of us can't.*
>
> Andrea

Andrea acknowledged her professional position, and that the task, however distasteful, must be completed. There was an intermingled sense of acceptance with an important honest acknowledgement that, given the option, Andrea would rather someone else dealt with the baby whose skin was macerating. There was an empathic understanding of why some of her colleagues distance themselves from these situations.

For many years it has been considered good midwifery practice to support the mother in seeing and holding her stillborn infant (Too 1995; Foster 1996). Such a sad task is made worse when the baby's body is less than normal in appearance. In Ann's account the mother was clearly reluctant to view her child; undeterred, the midwife attempted once again to try and make things better, while acknowledging that she had been in worse situations. Ann's long pause and removal of eye contact reinforced that she was comparing past experiences; her smile confirmed that she had seen much worse-looking stillborn babies, and that given the opportunity she could make the child more presentable.

> *We did not dress her immediately, Dad was cuddling her, but Mum didn't touch her at all; the baby was macerated but not that bad. Her colour was pretty good really; she was not black like some of the others! Her skin was peeling in parts, she had only just started to go off. She looked quite nice really and . . .* (long pause, looks down then up, smiles and looks down again) *I knew that if I took her away I could make her nicer looking.*
>
> Ann

Despite professional and hospital policies that direct the midwife to encourage parents to hold their dead baby, such encouraging of bereaved parents to view, hold and bond with their dead baby is not always an easy task (Mander 2006; Boyle 1997; Hockey, Katz and Small 2001). Some couples need no encouragement to hold their baby and view it like any other; others need support and encouragement to take that arduous and emotionally painful step.

> *I said to her, 'he looks like you' and she burst into tears and I thought 'should I have said that or should I not' and I thought, 'well I said his face is perfect.'* (smiles very slowly) . . . *I said 'you could just look at him and hold his hand; you don't have* (emphasises the word 'have') *to hold him' and then I left again and that afternoon she decided to see him but her partner never did* (shakes her head slowly).
>
> Claire

Since this data was collected, policy has changed on this matter and midwives are now required to give 'sensitive support' in offering mothers the choice of whether to see and hold their dead baby (NICE 2010). Such facilitation of choice for a grieving mother is another demanding emotional labour for midwives. If the mother does not wish to hold her dead baby, the midwife has to support her in the present while also considering the parents' possible future regrets if they choose not to see or hold their baby.

Verbal interaction must continue during the immediate hours post delivery as procedures and policies are finally completed and, as these accounts verify, during that time the parents may make requests of the midwife that she may not later be able to fulfil. An issue emerged that became entitled 'professional lies'; it serves to highlight that sometimes the midwife's belief and value system may be challenged as a decision must be made as to where and with whom her professional time must now be given.

PROFESSIONAL LIES

Interwoven in the communication between the mother and the midwife is a small, but significant, pattern of professional lies, apparently used as a means of supporting the mother in the overall desire to make things better. Professional lies may be condoned as commendable actions by some individuals; conversely, others would consider that they are unacceptable, unethical and contrary to the midwives' professional code of practice (NMC 2008).

When a loved one dies, close relatives are invariably highly sensitive to what is going to happen to the body. Requesting permission for a post mortem examination or being told that one is being sought is an emotional and difficult experience to cope with and must not be underestimated as to its impact (Dickinson, Johnson and Katz 2000). The activity of having to request parental signature for a post-mortem examination, and finally having to wrap a child's body in plastic with identification tags and placing them in a suitcase-like structure is not an enviable task for any midwife or neonatal/paediatric nurse.

Following a death, the grieving relatives must trust that their loved one's body will be treated with respect by healthcare workers. Parents of stillborn babies are anxious to ensure the safe conveyance of their baby's body to the hospital mortuary. However, sometimes promises made to the parents by the midwife for varying reasons were not kept and some midwives resorted to telling professional lies. A possible explanation for Kathryn's and Ann's actions may be that they were in a state of dissonance or conflict regarding allocation of their time. The narratives show their ability to reflect and rationalise their actions positively and, in doing so, free themselves from negative emotions. The non-verbal communication of a series of large smiles reinforced their spoken opinion. They felt that it was acceptable, under certain circumstances, to receive gratitude from parents and to simultaneously seek to mislead them, rather than upset them further by explaining that there were new priorities now on the midwife's time.

I always say to them when I am taking the baby away that this is the final thing and that the baby is going away now and you are going to the ward . . . I cannot say I am not taking the baby to the mortuary; I lie to them and say I will carry it down and I will look after it just the way that I am looking after it now (smiles broadly).

Kathryn

Their faces just light up (smiles broadly) *and they say, 'thank you for bathing and taking the baby'* (big broad smile). *I tell a very little lie* (long pause). *I lie because I know I do not have the time to take it away from the delivery suite when we are busy, and so I get a porter to take it but they do not know that.*

Ann

I feel quite comfortable at telling them that little white lie and quite often when I get cards back it quite often says that 'it helped knowing that you were taking James over to the mortuary' and I thought they were happy thinking that it was being looked after right up to the end. That is fine I think? (Smiles again and nods at me.)

Susanna

The examples presented above of professional lies are all linked to events where both the mother and the midwife knew that an intrauterine death had occurred. In the case of Sophie, a community midwife, tragedy struck while she was conducting a home birth. This community midwife, the mother and family were all prepared for the arrival of a healthy baby. Unfortunately, the infant was stillborn due to an abnormality, which was incompatible with extrauterine life. In this unique account regarding an unpredicted tragedy, the midwife concerned made a decision that may or may not be seen as ethically acceptable by her professional peers. Sophie was resolute that her professional lie made things a little better for the woman in a state of shock.

She said she held me in no way responsible for anything that had happened and was very grateful for allowing her to have a hug goodbye – was pleased I'd let the baby die in her arms because she firmly believed that she'd been holding her baby when it died . . . We . . . knew it hadn't.

Sophie

Communication with individuals at the time of a death is never an easy task. Saunders and Valente (1994) identify that nurses, after sudden deaths, often experience relentless self-questioning around their own professional beliefs, values and moral obligations. It is arguable that Sophie considered it was morally right for the mother to believe that she had given birth within her home to a live baby who unfortunately could not sustain life.

In this study, the 12 midwives mirrored the findings in the studies of Saunders and Valente (1994), Lamers (1997), Rashotte, Fothergill-Bourbonnais and Chamberlain (1997) and Cutler (1998) in that they are seen to function from bereavement frameworks constructed from their own experiences around loss. The issue of 'shedding a tear' and showing emotion is revisited to examine how it is linked to the midwife's professional image. In this context, it embraces issues regarding communication at the time of the stillbirth; the shedding of tears is seen as means of conveying to the parents the midwife's personal feelings surrounding the event.

SHEDDING A TEAR AND SHARING THE LOSS

The literature concerning the impact of the death of patients on nurses and midwives often raises the issue of whether they should show emotions in front of relatives. Over half of the midwives considered that shedding a tear and removing the professional mask was a natural human response, and that it communicated to the mother that they too were saddened by the event. Hockey, Katz and Small (2001) consider that healthcare professionals are often reluctant to be seen to legitimise and communicate their true feelings at times of death. When the midwives tried to communicate their feelings they did so amidst an air of confusion, fuelled by labile periods of rationalisation, and then internalised conflict. Self-criticism surfaced despite reassurance given to them by some mothers that the midwife's emotional communication was perceived as a comfort and indicated that the loss of her baby had meaning to others also.

Too (1995) writes that there can never be a policy on crying and no predetermined emotional response. All the midwife can do is to take cues from the individual parents and respond accordingly. Lovell (1986) states that, in her experience, mothers often express their appreciation of those midwives who cared so much that they cried with them. Such statements seek to emphasise the variable depths of connection between the mother and her midwife. Defey (1995) is of the opinion that emotions are bound to run high as death is a painful thing to watch, and that crying is an open expression of the shock and grief of the situation and is a legitimate response. Parkes (2002) writes of the importance of everyone operating from a secure base, existing amongst individuals who encourage the expression of feelings. These following quotations succinctly identify the internal conflict on this issue that some midwives experienced.

> Yes I cry, it's so painful when it happens . . . I've been around a long time; we don't talk about emotions.
>
> Becky

> I always cry, can't help myself.
>
> Janet

> I think they think you're hard if you don't cry. It's the little things, like you just go up to them . . . touch the hand and say 'I'm here, I'm here to look after you, here to support you' and no, I don't think it's professional weakness because I think you're human – to me human . . . don't be frightened to cry.
>
> Linda

> I am quite an emotional person, I shed tears easily . . . I cry as I am delivering these women. There is nothing shocking about showing these women that you are sorry for them . . . but sometimes, yes I wonder am I doing the right thing you know.
>
> Lesley

In the accounts of some respondents there was also indecisiveness concerning crying with the parents. However, they differ in that they make brief but important admissions that in retrospect could have been further explored had a second interview taken place after primary data analysis. There is the acknowledgement that parents have told them of their awareness that their stillbirth may have affected them emotionally as the attending midwife. This highlights the importance of recognising the varying connections between some mothers and their known midwife at these times.

I did not cry at the time, but when the mother thanked me I couldn't stop crying . . . look at me I am crying now! (Laughing and crying simultaneously so the tape is stopped.)

Susanna

I always cry always, not at the same point, but at some stage, I always cry with the parents I don't know if it is appropriate . . . I started to cry and I said to her 'I know it's hard, I know it's hard' . . . but they say to me, 'it must be awful for you too' . . . But I do . . . yes I do have many doubts.

Kathryn

Is it appropriate? . . . I find myself asking that . . . but mothers say 'it must be awful for you too', they pat my hand and they think I am human . . . and at the end of the day you are, you cannot help but cry and it does show that you are grieving.

Claire

Oh! No, No I do not think it is wrong for the midwife under such circumstances to cry. The crying of staff sometimes helps the mothers, for I have spoken to mothers who have had stillbirths and they say that it helps them when staff show emotion. It helps, but sometimes even the mothers say they feel guilty because they see themselves as being the cause of the sadness. That can sometimes, I feel, be dreadful because the loss is theirs but . . . (long pause) *so many have said that they appreciate that we suffer the loss with them . . . so many keep in touch.*

Andrea

Andrea's account shows the complexity of this issue. Clearly the midwife must manage her expression of emotion so as to respond as she feels will help the mother and it must not just be a spontaneous or routine expression of her own sadness. Defey (1995) argues that the sight of a distressed midwife who is emotionally reacting to a tragic scene may compound the negative impact on the parents, and that the midwives' displays of emotion in some instances may generate further feelings of culpability within the mother. The mother may consider that she is not only responsible for the loss of her baby, but also the feelings of the midwife. Andrea is aware of this, but is still of the view that crying with the mother is acceptable, as is the need to maintain connection with her.

Communication with the mother was in some instances prolonged after the stillbirth and beyond the midwives' professional requirement to attend to the mother. This prolongation of communication and personal contact between the midwife and the mother was present in over half of the 12 narratives despite acknowledgement of the emotion that pervaded such meetings or periods of contact. Similar findings were reported by Rashotte, Fothergill-Bourbonnais and Chamberlain (1997), Lamers (1997), Wright (1998) and Gardner (1999).

KEEPING IN TOUCH

It is normal professional practice for community midwives, when satisfied with the mother's and baby's progress, to discontinue care after the tenth postnatal day. Midwives who maintained contact with bereaved parents or relatives saw this as an enabling activity, which allowed them to find ways of handling their own grief around the death while also supporting the bereaved parents. Attending funerals appeared to have provided two community midwives with the opportunity to seek closure to the event and to disengage themselves from the family and professionally move on, while at the same time being seen to pay their respects to the mother and her family. It was considered significant, therefore, that none of the hospital-based midwives spoke of attending funerals as an opportunity to engage in a cathartic experience.

Sonia was seen to reflect for several seconds and question herself as to her reasons for attending funerals. Her non-verbal communication was congruent with her spoken words: she looked sad as she acknowledged that, like the parents of the baby, she was experiencing painful emotions. There was heavy emphasis on the word 'hurting' but also acknowledgement of the important support that was present within her midwifery team. Sonia, and especially Linda, placed great emphasis on their own personal decision to attend the funerals and there was no sense of professional coercion.

> *I think she thought she could talk to me. I used to go, and it used to be an hour's visit or more. It wasn't a problem because she could talk to me . . . she knew she could talk to me. I did all the visits and we were ready to discharge her but I didn't discharge her until the twenty-eighth day, she wouldn't let me go . . . Yes, but because I knew what I wanted too, I felt I wanted to do it . . . I go to all the funerals.*

Linda

> *We go to the babies' funerals as a team whenever possible or, at least two or three of us to support each other.* (Her head goes down then she looks up to the ceiling then back to the interviewer.) . . . *Yes I do I really do* (nods head repeatedly), *I think that it's like . . .* (very, very long pause). *It's like you have known them as a person that couple . . . you know what's happened and it is about showing your mark of respect to them, and to tell, just tell them that we are hurting too.*

Sonia

Communicating with one unfortunate woman over a prolonged period of time, following a stillbirth, became extremely problematic for Andrea, who was also coming to terms with the death of her own father. In trying to meet the emotional needs of the mother, Andrea's willingness to step outside her professional boundaries impeded her ability to disengage from the mother professionally and personally. Andrea later became aware that the woman required care beyond her scope of professional practice, but she did not have the knowledge or skill to refer the woman at that time. The ability to understand when to refer a bereaved mother to her GP for psychological assessment is clearly important.

She was phoning me at home . . . I realised she was not just keeping in touch with me to talk about what had happened but because she wanted to keep links with me as a friend.

Andrea

Grieving mothers may not be alone in needing reassurance and reinforcement of their self-esteem. A midwife may equally need reassurance herself. The three accounts below show a very strong desire to have feelings validated by a special person, not a colleague but, in these instances, the mother of the child. Further evidence of a degree of connection between a mother and her known midwife emerged.

I wanted to do it, support her . . . she did not want me to go . . . she did not want me to stop going . . . it felt good to me that she felt I was the one who could help her . . . It got to the case of the more you do the more you get into it, and I used to find it rewarding to a certain extent, because the women were usually so grateful (large smile on her face).

I remember talking to her afterwards . . . she said, 'thank you' to me and said she knew that I did all that I could.

Linda

Through critical analysis of herself, Sonia was able to justify expressing her personal needs. Having her needs met allowed Sonia to find closure to the stillbirth experience and to realign her relationships; she sought to conclude the experience as a person who did all she could. Sonia's head and eye movements confirmed that she was reflecting and allowing memories to surface. The smile that later appeared was interpreted as Sonia acknowledging her personal needs, which some people may find unacceptable.

Oh yes definitely, I wish I had seen her again . . . I am thinking now why (puts her head back and looks up at the ceiling) *. . . Doreen, for very selfish reasons if I am honest, I feel that I would have . . . it's about . . . well it's about justifying yourself to be honest. I wanted to hear from her about how she felt about things and I wanted her to say to me . . . 'you did all that you could' . . . that is just what I wanted to hear her say, which I know is purely selfish* (smiles broadly).

Sonia

Death had a profound impact on the professional and personal lives of these midwives. The midwife's role will always be a creative one, responding to the individual mother, and in tragic events such as stillbirth, midwives must learn to manage their own emotions so as to support the mother without becoming too overtly involved with their client's tragedy. This activity requires midwives to have the necessary skills to disengage themselves effectively.

This study has shown that communicating at the time of a stillbirth is a complex activity. Channels of communication may be difficult to sustain, while there is equally a strong desire at times for both the midwife and the mother to communicate specific needs. Some midwives needed the woman's confirmation that they had done all that they could professionally, given the tragic circumstances. The mother's acknowledgement was important in influencing the ability of the midwife to cope with and learn from the stillbirth.

CHAPTER 7

Taking the blame and feeling the guilt

Feelings of anger, blame and guilt are common manifestations of the grief process. Individuals who are party to, or have witnessed, a traumatic event may express emotions that may be unleashed on and towards a multitude of individuals for a variety of reasons; for example, towards a person seemingly not valuing the physical and emotional lives of the bereaved (Weston, Martin and Anderson 1998). Equally, strong emotions may be focused on the self for seemingly failing an individual, as feelings of guilt and self-reproach are often focused upon something that happened or was felt to be neglected around the time of the death (Worden 2003; Figley, Bride and Mazza 1997).

A sense of outrage following several of the stillbirths was evident in the words and the non-verbal communications of the midwives. Some showed great insight into the parents' need to blame, but dealing with their own blame responses was difficult in their work culture and in the absence of formal support structures.

These findings fit with the research of Cutler (1998), Wakefield (2000) and Payne (2001) in that healthcare workers have difficulty coming to terms with loss when they work in an atmosphere of professional conflict, blame and criticism, even when no evidence of culpability is present. Worden (2003) suggests that blame, guilt and anger around loss arise from a sense of frustration around the constant speculation as to the preventability of the death.

TAKING THE BLAME: SHE HAD A RIGHT TO BLAME SOMEONE

For the midwives interviewed, self-blame concerning the death was common. This was exacerbated by and closely linked with their feeling that blame was inevitable and, as professionals, they could expect to be blamed by relatives of the dead baby and they should accept that blame.

It is common practice for community, if not hospital, midwives to attend the funeral of a stillborn baby when they have cared for the mother. In the view of two community midwives attendance at these funerals created the opportunity, not only to convey their own and their colleagues' condolences, but to present an unsaid apology or acceptance of the blame for professionally letting the couple down. Andrea's level of disquiet was particularly evident as she placed great emphasis on certain words relating to feelings and culpability. Her body language confirmed her anxiety; her hands tightly gripped the microphone and her body posture changed from being relaxed to being rigid.

> *It's about showing your mark of respect to them. It is also to say you know* (pause) *we hurt; we feel* (great emphasise made, clenches hands on to the microphone). *Have we let you down, have we done anything? . . . but we are still here for you, if and when you need us . . . Because you do blame, you do blame yourself, oh yes, you do blame yourself in these awful situations because of the circumstance.*
>
> Andrea

Being the recipient of parental and family outbursts of anger was rationalised by two of the midwives as the relatives having a legitimate right to blame someone for their loss. Such rationalisation showed insight into the grieving process, an understanding that people in grief display a wide spectrum of emotional and cognitive responses. Yet, even with such insight, it is difficult to cope with receiving the anger and blame of an individual who is shocked and bewildered following a sudden death.

Claire was aware that taking such blame may not be the right response, yet felt she should do this, despite her own pain.

> *We take the blame you know, we know we shouldn't but we do . . . this father-in-law was shouting at me, he was grieving, but I felt he was right to shout at me. You know, but I was feeling all these painful things.*
>
> Claire

Becky's exaggerated head movements, and her raised vocal tone on the word 'you' conveyed the awfulness of the situation.

> *The lady's husband was almost fainting in the corridor . . . the woman's father is shouting and poking me and saying, 'we brought my daughter into you last night. We were worried about the baby's movements, we did all we should but you, you let our baby die' . . . I had to take this hell!* (Shakes and nods her head violently.)
>
> Becky

Self-blame and acceptance of the blame of others arises in the accounts of a further three midwives, who saw such blame as inevitable. Other respondents reassured themselves that no amount of cajoling by colleagues, not even if they were correct, could dismiss their grief.

> *It just does not matter what people say to you afterwards, it is that feeling of guilt and blame that you are always* (puts flat of hand down on to her knee) *. . . left with, you*

always are. We all have to blame somebody for letting this happen to us . . . Just what a waste, what a waste, she surely had a right to blame somebody! (Very long pause . . . still looking out of the window.) *I had spent such a long time checking things, but . . .* (long pause again) *. . . I still think that I had the responsibility. I felt responsible.*

Andrea

When I saw her I felt so guilty, guilty that we had allowed this to happen even though we could not have stopped it.

Janet

The horror the guilt . . . (long pause) *. . . staff – they were saying to other colleagues, the team, and me . . . that I had done all that I could . . . the mother did not impart any blame on to me. However, I still feel some blame . . . could I have acted quicker?*

Linda

Sonia acknowledged feelings of unproven culpability. She was adamant that the stillbirth was not only preventable but that she was personally culpable in some way. In addition, she uses the word 'they' and 'we' to blame herself and her medical colleagues.

The FH just went and we lost the baby, all because they failed to act . . . I failed to act . . . I failed . . . We failed.

Sonia

Feelings of blame fused with anger surrounding loss, if not directed somewhere, may be turned inward, resulting in depression, guilt, or lowered self-esteem (Worden 2003). These midwives reported no support in finding ways to defuse their anger and realign their own levels of personal control.

The need for support and guidance in reflection, following a traumatic event, is particularly clear in the narrative of one community midwife. Sophie's description of a sudden stillbirth contains elements of anger, disbelief, numbness, shock and a subsequent lowering of self-esteem. All of these emotions are encapsulated in a numbing acceptance of the finality of her situation and the blame that she has to bear. Of all the 12 interviewees, this midwife exhibited the least variation in non-verbal communication, and yet Sophie's experience was considered to be the most deeply disturbing and reflective narrative in this study. She displayed complete composure; she sat erect throughout the interview, making only occasional eye contact to confirm that I was listening, and stayed looking straight ahead into the garden. (Such rigid body language simultaneously emphasised the importance and the difficulty of maintaining appropriately responsive body language as the researcher.) Sophie maintained her total self-composure for the 45 minutes of the interview.

Weston, Martin and Anderson (1998) consider that some people can be deeply upset and disorientated by changes that death brings about in their life's routine.

Such shock and resulting changes may not be immediately evident at the time of the death but like shock waves, they resonate for variable lengths of time. In Sophie's account there is a strong sense of her taking the blame that encompasses numerous losses. The stillbirth had devastating reverberations for her and she later explained that she considered her losses to be more than just the baby. She identified her lost connection with the mother; loss of her own sense of normality; and, most importantly, loss of her professional integrity, self-worth and self-esteem. This acknowledgement of multiple losses was vocalised after the tape recorder was turned off, but Sophie gave full approval for them to be described within this study.

In this extract Sophie pronounced herself guilty without trial and her sense of culpability was overwhelming.

> *I believed I'd let the baby die. I was totally responsible for this death* (long pauses between her words). *I was devastated – but didn't question their judgement in making any decision about me, I accepted it totally. I had let a baby die . . . that [suspension from my work] was the right thing to do because I was not a competent practitioner. I didn't need help from anybody else to believe that I wasn't a competent practitioner . . .* (very long pause; breathing heavily) . . . *I not only felt I had let a baby die . . . in fact I totally believed it . . . I and only I was responsible.*

Sophie

This midwife's shock and disbelief was evident; however, there was no questioning of the decision made to suspend her, possibly due to her feelings of numbness. This shows how, given the right antecedents, a midwife may, like the mother, exhibit the same first stage of grief – blame – as described by Kubler-Ross (1970), Parkes (1996, 1998) and Worden (2003). As for the mother, a midwife's emotional healing may be sabotaged by an inability to initiate self-forgiveness, even with, as in this case, proven exoneration from a district coroner that no action on this midwife's part could have changed the outcome.

The perpetuation of self-blame can be a harmful maladaptive response to loss, for it has the ability to undermine feelings of self-worth and can keep the individual entrenched in a sense of profound negativity. Some of the midwives continued to feel that they must be to blame; others could move on from self-admonishment to assessing the whole situation.

> *The consultant came on and played hell about this baby, I felt like I had killed a baby . . . but then I thought, 'why the hell is she playing hell with me' . . . she wrote the guidelines that I had stuck to . . . it didn't help me at the time but now it does . . . I can see that I was a pawn in a sequence of events.*

Becky

Andrea's narrative contains evidence of reflection and analysis of her actions and the actions of others at the time. The big smile at the end of this telling, coupled with her spoken words, conveys a strong sense of resolution and deep personal relief.

At first I felt like I had caused that death to occur, I should have bypassed the registrar and gone straight to the consultant. Then I thought, 'no, the registrar had a responsibility to contact the consultant' . . . *but for a long time I held the guilt, thinking, 'what did the woman think of me?'* . . . *but* (smiles broadly) *not now* . . . *no more!*

Andrea

I felt powerless . . . *angry at that doctor* . . . *we lost a baby and I did not know why* . . . *then I started to think, you know Doreen, some stillbirths cannot be explained; you just have to reflect on that.*

Sally

Through the process of realigning their feelings of guilt and the re-establishing of personal control, some of these midwives achieved a degree of resolution. Worden (2003) identifies that, through exploration with the individual, the anger surrounding 'Why didn't I do this or that?' could be brought to a resolution of 'I suppose I did all that I could under the circumstances'.

Defey (1995) is of the opinion that feelings of guilt and blame are intrinsically linked to both personal and professional loss of control and anger at the situation healthcare workers may find themselves embroiled in. This was seen in the accounts of several of the midwives, where a strong sense of blame and anger associated with individuals and events came through in an impassioned manner. The pervading sense of blame was unwarranted and even though the midwives appeared to rationalise that the blame was not attributed to them, nevertheless, as an emotion it remained, as can be seen in the words of Sonia and Lesley.

Ummm . . . *again I delivered this baby and I have always been angry about it and* . . . *I have never been able to resolve it* (heavy emphasis on the words; face alters and right hand is put into a fist shape). *I have just never been able to resolve the anger I have about it. The reason being that I got the job* (points finger in to her own chest) *of having to deliver this lovely big fat healthy boy, who was dead* . . . *I wasn't to blame!*

Sonia

As with most survivors of a death or tragic event, the search for a cause or someone to blame is relentlessly pursued, even if it that leads to them blaming themselves (Figley, Bride and Mazza 1997; Weston, Martin and Anderson 1998).

I got called out of my room by the coordinator to go and scrub in theatre for a section and I said 'I can't I have got my lady who needs me!!' (Strong emphasis on her words) . . . *I was shouted down you know. She said* . . . *'I need you!'* (Emphasis on the 'you'.) *'You will go and do it'* (holds hands together tightly on lap, face alters, mouth tightens). *I had no time to go in and explain to her* . . . *and I had this intense feeling that when that woman needed me the most I was not there for her!*

Lesley

Sonia's and Lesley's facial and bodily gestures served to reinforce and display their anger, and in that anger, feelings of guilt and blame became intertwined with feelings of loss of control. There are parallels between the accounts of Sonia and Lesley on several levels: they both experienced frustration around having lost control of their immediate practice, as well as that practice being undermined by self-blame.

In Lesley's situation, from the viewpoint of management, the needs of the woman requiring an emergency delivery were far more important than the needs of the mother with the intrauterine death whose labour was progressing normally. Yet that mother then suffered another loss: that of the midwife who was supporting her. Causing the mother that further loss resulted in Lesley feeling anguish; anger at herself and others was over-ridden by an overwhelming sense of blame at having failed the client she related to as 'my lady'. Though required to take on the additional work, she accepted the blame she could have attributed to management.

My own experience (DK) of tragedy both personally and professionally confirms the theory that survivors, be they relatives or as in this study, midwives, often retrace their steps leading up to and around the time of the death (Kubler-Ross 1970; Worden 2003; Parkes 1996).

> *I spent a long time, re-checking things, but I still think that I was to blame.*
>
> Sally

> *It all seemed such a blur . . . but I kept going over it and checking things.*
>
> Sonia

> *I remember going over and over the guidelines, checking had I done things right.*
>
> Becky

> *I checked everything, went back and did it again.*
>
> Sophie

Feelings of guilt are clearly present in these accounts. Those negative feelings had an impact not only on the midwives as individuals, but also on their perceived professional image.

FEELING THE GUILT: PROFESSIONAL FAILURE

Feelings of anger and guilt associated with death are a normal reaction to loss (Kubler-Ross 1970; Hockey, Katz and Small 2001). Other studies show that health-care workers' feelings of guilt focus on a sense of culpability. Weinberg (1995) states that mourners who blame themselves often try the hardest to make some amends. Severe remorse is seen most frequently around the deaths of young children and babies (Rashotte, Fothergill-Bourbonnais and Chamberlain 1997; Hockey, Katz and Small 2001), since age is one variable that is used to classify a death as a meaningful event. Associated feelings of guilt were described by most midwife respondents.

The feelings of guilt expressed by the midwives were often still labile and unpredictable after a long interval. The midwives were seen to have dispersed their guilt and anger over a wide range of issues. This dispersal of anger and the targeting of guilt is a normal reaction to bereavement and is part of the feelings associated with the trauma of grief (Figley, Bride and Mazza 1997; Worden 2003). According to Figley, Bride and Mazza (1997), a stressor capable of producing trauma usually evokes feelings of intense fear, helplessness, guilt or horror. The word 'horrible' is one that the midwives themselves linked to personal feelings of guilt at the time of the stillbirth. The feelings of guilt present in these accounts are illuminated further by the midwives' non-verbal communications. These accounts are from midwives working in all areas of clinical practice.

> *It is always a difficult situation but when I look back it always fills me with sadness and the funny thing is, the most guilt . . . if someone has a stillbirth and I've been directly involved with their care, this is just horrendous, so horrible.*
>
> Ann

> *Suddenly* (very long pause), *I recalled the event and my guilt came flooding back . . . it was so horrible. Then they thanked me for the care I had given, and I felt even more guilty . . . it was horrible, just horrible.*
>
> Susanna

Kathryn also experienced guilt feelings that were deeply felt and revisited.

> *Oh that guilt trip I had . . . was horrible, just so horrible* (starts to cry; tape is stopped).
>
> Kathryn

Recounting those memories appeared to also reactivate the emotions Kathryn felt at the time and she became very emotional. This was apparent in several other narratives.

> *Through professional experience I realise that I am not over the top, or on a fine line, everybody is like that, it is this awful feeling of horror and guilt.*
>
> Becky

> *We all do our best on the antenatal unit, but I think of these women often and I feel so guilty . . . so guilty.*
>
> Janet

> *You do your best . . . you do blame yourself for the circumstances, you do blame yourself for the situation . . . I felt so very guilty and no matter what . . . psychologically and emotionally it is quite a burden.*
>
> Sonia

I remember talking to her (the mother) *afterwards really so to speak to get over my own guilt trip . . . I did not want her babies to go in the sluice . . . we needed a bereavement room then. I remember thinking we should all have been stronger, and got things changed a long time before.*

Susanna

Defey (1995) acknowledges the ease with which guilt feelings develop in staff that have to deal with infant deaths, with a resulting transference of feelings of anger on to other colleagues who may or may not have been party to the events. A strong sense of anger and agitation, both verbal and non-verbal, emanated from the midwives during the narrations.

I was absolutely drained and while I was washing the baby the midwife in charge of the ward said did I want any help? I said no but she sent in an auxiliary nurse that was quite aggressive . . . I had had a do with her! . . . Oh no, not the best person to send to me . . . so I told her to go, and leave me to it (looks angry).

Sonia

I met that doctor again! . . . I thought 'that woman!' (Pursed lips and frowning.) *I looked straight at her and I am sure she recognised me . . . that woman walked into the room and I looked at her and thought . . . 'I can't believe it' . . . I just could not deal with what I felt* (face looks angry).

Sally

You feel this anger and you just want to put it somewhere, anywhere (shakes her head and makes a fist) *. . . I felt so angry when the doctor said, 'I will come after my lunch . . . but if you are worried get someone else to see her' . . . I just felt sick.*

Becky

Claire was the only midwife who felt she was deliberately subjected to another colleague's black humour or displaced negative feelings (*see* Recrimination by colleagues, pp. 102–3).

Stillbirth cases are reviewed by obstetricians, paediatricians and midwives at regular perinatal mortality meetings. The primary aim of these meetings is to discuss individual cases in-depth, consider the overall clinical management, review hospital policies and procedures, and discuss staff educational requirements. These meetings can be 'extremely useful' provided that they are 'conducted in a non-judgemental atmosphere' (Magowen, Owen and Drife 2009; 391). However, the midwives interviewed felt that attending a perinatal mortality meeting created tension and a defensive stance amongst all those present. A midwife must accept that every facet of her practice will be analysed by the meeting and subjected to professional scrutiny. Yet Andrea viewed the perinatal mortality meeting as a trial, and only when she had been tried and found not guilty would she allow herself permission to seek personal closure to the tragic event. Susanna and Sally also found the meeting threatening and likened it to 'going into battle'.

> *It is taking the scenario further . . . for it's the perinatal mortality meeting when every-thing is scrutinised. You feel like you are defending yourself* (points finger repeatedly into her chest); *it is the third degree, for they are looking critically at everything, where and when was this baby compromised? So it is not a blame-free culture. I took a copy of everything . . . cos things change and I felt like I was going into battle . . . I felt like the doctors were trying to lay the blame on me . . . I felt awful for it seemed like, unknowing to the mother, there is a sideline battle . . . them and us, a sense of let's look after ourselves.*
>
> Andrea

> *Yes it is very threatening. I think there are a lot of things in midwifery that are very threatening because of the risk management side. Risk management side is support-ing a blame-free culture and to learn from happenings, because there are good things as well as bad things which come out of situations and we don't seem to focus on the good, it is always on the negative really . . . it's like going into battle.*
>
> Susanna

> *It's looked at as strict policing, dissecting notes, not a debriefing session . . . no chew-ing the fat . . . which is what in reality is needed . . . it can be very threatening those meetings . . . but things are better now that supervision has changed; at least that is less threatening.*
>
> Sally

Within 24 hours of attending the stillbirth, Sophie was accused of professional malpractice and suspended from duty. It was to be days before that accusation was withdrawn. She then had to endure a verbal cross-examination and critical review of her case notes by her senior midwifery supervisor and later the district coroner's officer.

> *They, them . . . the managers dissected my notes and decided immediately that I had not practised appropriately . . . I had failed to resuscitate the baby and . . . I had failed to countersign my student's records . . . things had been ok and I thought I would do it at the end of the day . . . then in shock I forgot . . . in no state to return to practice . . . all this stuff was jumbled up in my head. The coroner's officer said I had let the baby die! I believed everyone . . . The coroner later exonerated me . . . I was not to blame, the baby had* (diagnosis not stated for reasons of confidentiality) *. . . it would never have survived.*
>
> Sophie

According to Worden (2003) most of the reasons given for the feelings of guilt and self-reproach are irrational, centring almost solely on the circumstances that lead up to the death. Sophie was judged to be guilty before all the evidence was collated. Not even exoneration at a level of investigation far above a perinatal mortality meeting could help her to disengage herself from the profoundly devastating impact of that experience. Fifteen years after that stillbirth, this midwife still sought resolution of the negative feelings she harboured towards others at that time. Sadly, no apology, formal counselling or support framework was available for her.

'SHEDDING A TEAR' AND SHOWING EMOTION

Weeping over a stillbirth was, for these midwives, closely linked with blame and the professional image of self and others expected and displayed at the time.

Each of us has feelings. We laugh and cry in our everyday lives. It is folly to expect us to wear a 'professional mask' to keep from displaying emotions within patient care settings (Lamers 1997: 63).

Wakefield (2000) considers that expressing grief is perceived as inappropriate by the wider professional bodies of healthcare practice. This is reinforced when society at large expects healthcare workers to be strong and resilient.

This study identified differing opinions amongst the midwives as to what constituted an appropriate professional image, and whether a midwife should be in emotional control whatever the circumstances. Seven of the midwives made direct reference to crying at the time of the stillbirth either in, or out, of sight of the woman, her partner and other colleagues. The issue of appropriate professional behaviour was closely linked with the midwives being fearful of saying or doing the wrong thing and this evoked further feelings of guilt within them. Internal conflicts surfaced, as the midwives appeared to experience a clash of personal beliefs and values.

> *You are only human you can't help but cry and it does show you are grieving, but is it appropriate? Is it appropriate for them to comfort you? I have my doubts. How professional can you be when you are crying in front of them, in front of the mum? They may not want you to cry.*
>
> Susanna

> *Because it's their grief, and I may be intruding on their grief, I may be distracting them and they might remember when they get home and say 'I was alright until the midwife started to cry and I couldn't cope then!'*
>
> Kathryn

> *The crying by the staff . . . well now, sometimes it helps the mothers, for I have spoken to mothers who had had stillbirths and they say that it helps them when staff show emotion . . . It helps but . . . then sometimes I wonder . . . the mothers may feel guilty because they see themselves as the cause of the sadness.*
>
> Andrea

I've always said when I've had a junior midwife with me or somebody who's not done a lot with people with stillbirths, 'don't be frightened to cry' . . . I don't think it is professional weakness, cause I think you're human to me, . . . yes, human.

Linda

The tensions around midwives' tears link personal needs for expression and protection with how they see their professional self (Cutler 1998; Wakefield 2000). While some of the midwives saw tears as a sign of being human, others were of the opinion that they should always display emotional control whatever the circumstances.

You are a professional person . . . you are expected to be strong . . . and we are very buttoned up, aren't we Doreen?

Sally

I never cry in public never . . . I pull myself together . . . I think midwives cannot talk about it, I think they feel it's theirs to hang on to within the hospital environment, they cannot inflict sorrow on other people.

Claire

I was well upset; I was welling up with tears, and yet it didn't seem appropriate you know . . . I don't know whether it's about trying to protect yourself and bottle things up.

Lesley

You've got to look strong and be strong . . . I remember thinking we should all be stronger.

Susanna

Anger and guilt for some of the midwives had additional roots in the words and facial expressions of other healthcare colleagues at the time of the stillbirth. Some midwives experienced negative verbal or non-verbal judgement at showing emotion in front of the couple. Others described recriminations and arguments over professional decision-making that impinged on their ability to obtain resolution to the experience. A small number of the midwives moved from a position of anger at their colleagues for their recriminatory remarks, to one of deep pervading resentment. Several of the midwives harboured deep anger towards colleagues whom they considered to be responsible for the death of the baby, and for placing them in either difficult or untenable professional positions.

RECRIMINATION BY COLLEAGUES

Four of the twelve midwives spoke of recrimination by doctors for what they saw as non-professional emotional behaviour. Lamers (1997) states that healthcare professionals, including doctors, must give each other permission to feel and grieve without fear of being rebuked. Parkes (2002) refers to everyone requiring a secure base from which to vent feelings during stressful times. The experiences of these midwives were very different.

Sonia disclosed her feelings concerning the doctor's recrimination for her not portraying an acceptable professional image. Her non-verbal communication showed that she was angry or disturbed by her recollections. When probed further, her anger erupted and she became clearly emotional.

> Sonia: *I delivered her, and I just felt beside myself, I felt so upset and so totally gutted. I felt so inadequate, and one of the doctors* (name withheld) *actually tore a strip off me . . . saying that I shouldn't be reacting!* (Tapping feet, looks agitated.)

> DK: *I am looking at your face now and can see you are disturbed.*

> Sonia: *Yes I am . . . I am a professional . . . but . . . I said 'I am only a human being!'* (Stressing the words and poking her finger into her chest.) *I felt so angry, so angry with* (name withheld). *I was in pain. I am also a human being and I also have feelings and I care . . . it was a case of stiff upper lip you know . . . I will never forget that.*
>
> Sonia

A similar experience was described by Janet, but for her there was the accusation, by the doctor present, that her display of emotion towards the mother after a diagnosis of intrauterine death was decidedly unhelpful. The outward display of emotion and what they saw as non-professional behaviour by the distressed midwife may have been difficult for the attending doctor to accept. Such lack of professional equanimity may have been perceived as threatening to the doctor's own professional composure.

> *I just went towards her and put my arms completely around her and she sobbed . . . I remember catching the eye of one of the doctors* (name withheld) *who was looking at me sternly as if to say 'pull yourself together'* (points finger inwards) *. . . [they] began verbally berating me and suggesting that I was not helping her at that time.*
>
> Janet

These two midwives described their feelings at comments passed by medical colleagues. A third midwife recalled sarcastic comments from the duty doctor in the form of black humour. For this midwife, her memories of two stillbirths are, in part, linked to the comments of the doctor. While these hurtful comments were aimed at her, the midwife was able to reflect on the contents of the conversation. She considered that the doctor's humour was perhaps hiding his own anguish.

> *I've had to face it now and deal with it, but actually there were five stillbirths that I wasn't involved in, but two that I was, him and me . . . the doctor kept on saying, 'Oh no! She's on! The curse of the labour ward. Who's going to die today?' When I got home I thought about it, and I thought, 'gosh, you know somebody could have been*

really upset by that and not wanted to go on the labour ward again' (long pause) . . .
It hasn't affected me.

Claire

This midwife made a seemingly important final statement that the doctor's insensitive words had not affected her. However, the long pause that preceded that statement and lack of any eye contact with the researcher belied this, for the doctor's comments were clearly remembered and easily recalled.

Sonia described how tragic stillbirth events can lead to a midwife isolating herself and was of the opinion that any professional conflict at that time merely compounds that isolation. This midwife's comments support the opinion of McVicar (2003) in that professional conflict can undermine an individual's coping abilities in times of acute stress.

I will never forget what the doctor said to me (name withheld), *no sympathy just sarcasm and criticism . . . you can easily become isolated enough when this happens, you can easily cut yourself off, so you don't need them to do it to you!*

Sonia

These findings support those of Gardner (1999) and Wakefield (2000), who both describe their nurse respondents as not only coping with their own emotions and grief, but also experiencing insensitive comments from colleagues and physicians. In this study, several midwives considered that their professional culture was not one where they could approach a colleague and confront them with their displeasure or even anger and thereby enable emotions to be explored in a healthy and positive manner. Yet a professional culture that allowed the sharing of negative as well as positive feelings may go some way to facilitating personal and professional growth, albeit out of a tragic situation. To facilitate such exchanges would require both the medical and midwifery professions to confront issues of professional hierarchy. It would require all parties involved with stillbirths to be committed and open to providing a listening ear so that they may find resolution to their experiences around stillbirth.

CHAPTER 8

Listen to me, for we all need a degree of closure

Some stillbirths may render the midwife professionally saddened but require no closure other than the midwife recognising that all health professionals concerned acted appropriately. In such instances, at a suitable time, the professional ties with the mother cease and the midwife reinvests her professional skills and energy in other women, accepting that infant death does still occur despite advances in obstetric management.

Other stillbirths led midwives to display symptoms of acute grief for varying periods of time. The words 'listen to me, for we all need a degree of closure' are taken from the accounts of those midwives who sought to find ways to bring closure to memorable stillbirth events. While not on the scale of the parents' grief at bereavement, the initial shock and resulting disturbance to the physical and psychological equilibrium of the midwife in response to some stillbirths was clearly traumatic, as shown in previous chapters. A state of professional grief was clearly experienced and some of the respondents exhibited signs and activities that compared to the universal markers on bereavement and resolution of loss (Denzin and Lincoln 1998).

The literature on the need for reconciliation, closure or adjustment following loss (*see* Chapter 2), emphasises that, while we may all feel that we reach closure or resolution of loss by different means, the psychological markers that indicate movement towards this achievement are relatively constant (Worden 2003; Parkes 1996). In achieving closure on loss, bereaved individuals are often able to identify, on reflection, the precise time when they found that they could continue with their lives, both psychologically and socially. In this study, the midwives often knew what actions were required for them to move on, but being able or enabled to pursue that activity proved more difficult for some than for others.

Klass, Silverman and Nickman (1996) identify that seeking resolution to a death is as important as creating initial bonds and seeking ties to an individual or group: we can only seek resolution to that with which we have felt connected. The nature of the resolution of grief is intrinsically tied up with the nature of our bonds with the people concerned. Where midwives had developed relationships with clients over time, that relationship could create deeply felt loss if a stillbirth followed.

'Closure' may well not have been a good word to use in the context of this study. However, since the study was conducted using this word, we take it to mean 'obtaining a degree of acceptance of a situation, feeling comfortable with the memory because of performing well at the time and/or learning from the experience or absorbing the experience usefully into one's body of professional working knowledge'. In any of these senses, we see a degree of moving on from the experience, not forgetting it, but recycling the powerful emotions of the time so they empower learning but do not evoke feelings that have a negative impact on the individual when remembered.

THE NEED TO TALK

The individual's ability to articulate feelings, anxieties, and fears are cited in bereavement studies as making a significant contribution to achieving a state of acceptable closure or resolution around death and loss (Parkes 1996).

Ten of the twelve midwives interviewed had sought or were still seeking resolution to some of these tragic and traumatising events. Several of the midwives utilised their own support network, professional comradeship, immediate family members or close friends, to obtain a sympathetic listening ear. These midwives expressed a strong desire to talk about the stillbirth and its impact on them to a person accepted by them as sympathetic and with whom they felt a connection. Several said they wanted to talk with me (DK) because of my own experience of bereavement.

Talking with an appropriate person was an enabling activity that gave some of the respondents the ability to carry on functioning in their professional roles and, in some instances, in aspects of their personal lives. Sadly, several of the midwives felt professionally isolated, and had had little opportunity to convey their feelings when experiencing great anxiety.

For some midwives, the stillbirth left them with feelings of lack of control, guilt and professional depression that needed to be verbally expressed. This is highlighted by Becky.

> *I think it does help talking to people . . . it helps when people can anticipate how you feel . . . you can say 'did you have a swine of a night at home, has it affected your family?' Yes it helps but it's like this blackness . . . and it affects you . . . you're in a dark tunnel.*
>
> Becky

Though talking helps, Becky was aware that any midwife may have difficulty expressing their emotions verbally in these circumstances. She saw that the empathy of colleagues is helpful, especially when they have the skill to 'anticipate how you feel' and offer encouragement to talk. Claire used her own experience to do just that. Her assertive personality helped her talk openly about the issues she faced while caring for a woman with a stillbirth, and encouraged other midwives to relate their own experiences to her.

> *I just walked in and I talked straight away . . . everybody joined in and talked about a stillbirth that they'd had or dealt with and I think it probably did everybody good. Because everybody got their own experiences off their chests . . . I'm really talkative and I make talk and I ask questions and they all joined in and nobody seemed to get fed up with it, they were all happy to talk about it, went on for days. Well I think it was because they all came out with stories of their own experiences and they told it in huge detail, I think it was brilliant! I mean, a few of the midwives cried* (smiles and sits in an open posture).
>
> Claire

Claire understood from her previous experiences that few midwives spoke openly about their feelings around managing a stillbirth, and she decisively took on the role of a catalyst. Claire considered that her colleagues recounting their experiences and telling professional stories was 'brilliant' to behold.

In contrast, three midwives expressed a need to talk to colleagues about their experiences, but failed to grasp, or perhaps were not given, the opportunity. It may be that feelings of disbelief and numbness at that time stifled their ability to talk.

> *It is the sheer disbelief, you want to talk, but the words won't come out . . . yes on reflection now I realise that I did need to talk.*
>
> Susanna

The culture of NHS midwifery does not usually offer opportunities for such expression (Deery and Kirkham 2007). Critical reflection, albeit later, made several midwives aware that it would have been helpful to talk about the stillbirth and acknowledge the emotions that it engendered within them.

> *I do believe that I needed to talk then, yes we need to be encouraged to take the opportunity to talk . . . being encouraged to talk helps you to bring out your own grief . . . You put on a face because you are grieving for the mother and yourself.*
>
> Andrea

> *Midwives need to learn to talk; you need time to just be . . . you need to talk, even several days after the event you need to say how you are and what you feel.*
>
> Linda

Andrea was clearly aware of the nature of professional grief and she was resolute in her opinion that encouragement and opportunity for talk should be initiated by colleagues. Lack of such provision shows a neglect of the well-being of those providing a service, such as midwifery, where the need will inevitably arise. Yet this lack was experienced at an organisational and at an informal collegial level.

Recounting our experience is an enabling process that allows us to make sense of the events and feelings in our lives (Kirkham 1997; Wakefield 2000). Repeated telling provides the opportunity to reflect on events and their connotations, our role in them and to forge the story of that event, which allows us resolution of its immediate pain and admits the experience to the repertoire of professional stories on which clinical experience is built. The midwives needed to relate their stories of the tragic events in which they played a part; such a need resulted in them entering into this study. There was also a need to talk with the mother of the stillborn child.

EXPLAINING TO THE PARENTS

As well as a need to air their feelings, understand their experience and build their own stories, several midwives expressed a need to explain to the parents and thus influence their version of the story. They needed to talk with the mother and her partner following the stillbirth, to say how sorry they were and to discuss their part within the events or their apparent failure in some instances to keep promises because of other pressures upon them. Having the opportunity to converse and being able to convey their own feelings at the loss of the baby to the mother and her partner was seen as an essential start to obtaining closure on the experience. Talking with the parents and explaining why they were limited in the care they could give helped the midwives; and the parents' acceptance of these explanations played an important part in the midwives resolving their self-blame.

Weinberg (1995) hypothesises that making amends through verbal apology may help to promote recovery from the trauma experienced, as making amends is an enabling activity that is rooted in the belief that individuals operate in a just and morally ordered world. It is not possible to make amends for the death of a baby, yet seeking out the opportunity to explain and apologise helped individuals to reduce the deeply negative effects that are brought on by self-blame and lowered self-esteem, and limit the associated fear of further retribution.

Apology carries an acknowledgement of fault or failure, for English does not have a single word with which we can express our sadness and regret that something occurred without accepting blame. These midwives were English and the language, as well as the culture of the workplace, is likely to have influenced their response to tragedy.

Midwives are taught that they must always seek to maintain open channels of communication with clients and their families. Yet the organisation of care in the NHS involves many different carers and this fragmentation of care also fragments communication.

> As soon as you have sorted them out, and it can take a long time to sort them out . . . it's 'have you got that lady to the ward yet?', or 'have you arranged for that lady to go home?' . . . Yes, yes, unless they are staying on the delivery suite you end up with another lady and then they've gone and you can't get to talk to them and sort things out.
>
> Linda

Their need to say sorry and to inform the women that they did all that they could, given the tragic circumstance, was identified as motivating several of the midwives into considerable efforts to speak with the mothers at the earliest opportunity.

Lesley and Susanna described how that communication was also a hard task emotionally. Nevertheless, both midwives acknowledged a desire to make contact again with the women for some time after the stillbirth. In the development of both accounts a clear sense of urgency arose from their own emotional needs. It was they who had to initiate the reconnection and pursue dialogue with those women regarding the stillbirth.

> *The chance to discuss the events, a benefit for them as well as for your own . . . Yes it is*
> *. . . I suppose it is hard when for quite some time you feel that, you want to keep ring-*
> *ing up and pestering people by saying 'do you wish to see us or not?' When the time*
> *came for them to book again, they both came together, and they both agreed to see me*
> *. . . and it made such a difference talking about the stillbirth.*
>
> Lesley

> *You just try to get on with life and your job, but I wish we'd spoken to them. I cannot*
> *remember how long after, this mum came back with a full-term normal pregnancy.*
> *Then I thought, 'I just have to go and talk with her, just to ask if there is anything*
> *she wants to say to me, did she want to talk about things' . . . and we talked* (smiles,
> sighs then looks down on to her knees).
>
> Susanna

The smile at the end of the narration implies that Susanna was pleased that this meeting with the woman had been instigated and there is an unspoken acknowledgement that Susanna gained some degree of closure. However, the sigh and the removal of eye contact at the end of her narrative conveyed an air of sadness (Purtillo and Haddad 1996) that, for her, remained. Without such a meeting, closure is difficult.

> *I wish I had seen her again . . . I wanted her to say what I wanted to hear . . . I wanted*
> *her to say 'you did all that you could'.*
>
> Sonia

Hearing that acceptance of their efforts was part of the mother's story did a great deal to justify the midwife's story of the care she gave and her feeling that she was appreciated, despite the tragedy.

SEEKING OUT SUPPORT

To articulate negative feelings we often need support and permission from others (Worden 2003). The idea of the midwives requiring permission to articulate their feelings to others has arisen in earlier chapters of this book, especially with regard to bereaved parents. To receive or ask for the gift of support was seen by some of the midwives to impinge seriously on their professional image and served only to compound their intense and complex feelings of guilt. Several midwives experienced professional pain, feeling unsupported through lack of any acceptance by others of the intensity of their personal feelings.

A number of the midwives judged their degree of personal and professional support by whether their colleagues had encouraged discussion. The midwives appeared to need their colleagues to treat them, and all midwives, with congruence, unconditional regard and empathy in such dire events. These three qualities are the cornerstone for person-centred counselling (Egan 1990; Hockey, Katz and Small 2001). Congruence describes a state of operating within the parameters of honesty, and truthfulness to self. The need to display unconditional acceptance echoes the way in which being human was emphasised by the midwives as influencing how they responded to a stillbirth.

Seeking support from a particular group of colleagues was described by Lesley and Linda. They indicated that previous experiences with colleagues impacted on their decision as to whom they felt they could approach. Junior colleagues had preference over more senior ones, and yet it is with their senior colleagues that a wealth of comparable experience is likely to be found. Lesley suggested that some senior colleagues dismiss the emotions of others and were therefore not considered supportive.

> *It's a problem being on duty and wondering who can I seek that type of support from. It often tends to be probably junior colleagues, staff midwives that you are friends with . . . so you see how they* (points finger towards window) *react to situations and people think . . . 'no good asking her* (emphasis on the word 'her'). *If I was to ask her . . . for help or support she will just dismiss how I am feeling'.*
>
> Lesley

The social context of any encounter, including the perceived or known status of the people involved and the degree of friendship or perceived antagonism between them, affects the way in which individuals interpret a situation. This is clearly the case when midwives seek support within the hierarchical structures of the NHS, where the culture of midwifery expects self-sacrifice (Kirkham 1999) and asking for support or even a listening ear can be seen as a sign of weakness rather than professional insight. This is further complicated by the fact that the death of a baby is particularly distressing and is acknowledged to be a situation in which would-be supporters of bereaved individuals often fall by the wayside (Canine 1996).

Linda described how she alerted her support network that she was facing an intrauterine death and anticipated her subsequent feelings and support needs. Linda also clearly stated that not all colleagues were supportive; personal boundaries were often present that could not be encroached upon.

> *Well often when I have problems . . . I know who I can ring and say, and warn them in advance that they know something is going to happen . . . say, 'are you free tonight?' sort of thing* (smiles and giggles). *We miss out on getting that experience from certain*

people. I think it is there for the asking . . . (smiles) *if we ask for it* (great emphasis on the words) *. . . but it's about that line of knowing just how far to go you know!*

Linda

Worden (2003) is of the opinion that some people withdraw from friends perceived as being over solicitous and demanding of time and support; but within midwifery one would expect support needs to be reciprocated. Raphael (1996) sees care-eliciting actions as a form of attachment behaviour, which is normal when a human being is in emotional discomfort, but such activities reduce once the distress or threat to self starts to diminish.

Janet considered that care-eliciting behaviour was something to be encouraged. In her opinion such behaviour promotes the professional bonding or comradeship that is nurturing and protective towards colleagues facing an intrauterine death.

You can't really be prepared, but the unit that I'm in we're very supportive to each other. We look after each other with whatever happens and I'd just be asking if she is alright? Anything I could do to help in any way? and just to be aware, it is just so devastating.

Janet

Not all of the midwives sought support or indeed welcomed supportive gestures from colleagues. Becky considered her position as a senior midwife, and being a supervisor of midwives, left her without peer support. She felt that colleagues attempted to be supportive but this support arose from sympathy rather than empathy for they lacked her professional experience of stillbirths and this, together with her own motherhood status, affected her response to her colleagues' proffered support.

I was aware that my colleagues felt sorry for me (points her fingers into her chest), *cos they knew what had happened. I knew they were thinking, 'there but for the grace of God go I'. I knew it was said to make me feel better but it didn't. One very junior midwife said to me . . . 'Oh! I have never been involved in a tragedy', and that hurt me and I said 'well that's probably because you are inexperienced, cos the longer you do it the more you come into things.' That hurt me* (facial expression changes, no smile is present). *I think I was probably emotional because I'd got a baby as well.*

Becky

This study supports the proposals of Parkes (2002) and Canine (1996) which state that we all need a secure psychological base from which to function and the giving and receiving of support to verbalise personal feelings – in particular, those relating to the death of a child, are often clumsily offered and difficult to receive. The seeking of closure or the severing of emotional ties with these unfortunate mothers following their stillbirths may be considered an emotionally healthy activity that allows the midwife to reinvest her professional skills, time and energy in the direction of other pregnant women. Yet resolution to a loss requires an individual to reflect on her actions at the time of the event.

SEEKING CLOSURE OR RESOLUTION

There is little doubt that for these midwives many of the stillbirth events were emotionally painful and they sought to move on.

> *We all need a degree of closure don't we Doreen? . . . We need to move on.*
>
> Andrea

> *You do reflect on what's gone on, you see, you always, always wish that you could have done things better. Then you do know in truth you did your best . . . you did really.*
>
> Kathryn

> *You just get on with life . . . think about it a lot . . . and the job and then time just passes.*
>
> Susanna

Becky's experience and maturity, coupled with her ability to rationalise her professional position, helped her to understand how easy it would be to become a victim of circumstance. This attitude enabled her to move on.

> *It's difficult, as you know Doreen, you know you can't make it right for them so I try not to make myself feel like a victim, . . . I try to move on, the luck of the draw may make you feel like a victim but you're not really.*
>
> Becky

Andrea used the idea of unlocking the pain for the resolution of her professional grief. She acknowledged that failure to release herself from the pain of each stillbirth experience would prevent her from supporting other women and colleagues.

> *The pain is there and if you do not unlock it, when you are asked to support someone else going through it you are just not able to do it. Sometimes in cases like that you are not just grieving for the mother but also for yourself as well . . . so you are almost just not strong enough to cope with it.*
>
> Andrea

Funeral attendance can be an important stage in the resolution of loss. One community-based midwife saw attendance at funerals as a cathartic experience. Attending that final act of homage to the child, and saying goodbye to the parents enabled Sonia to find closure. Being present at the final death ritual helped her to close doors emotionally. She expressed the insight that closure or resolution following a death or loss is not something that one gives to individuals. It is noteworthy that these community midwives had relationships with their clients that had developed over time and they attended funerals as a team of trusted colleagues. Thus, they were supported to 'work through' their own process of grief resolution while offering their last support to the family.

We also now go to the funerals as a team . . . to support each other . . . I find it doesn't leave it all open in a way . . . I'm not very good at words here but it's about helping to finalise . . . you know what I mean Doreen, it's to sort of work through your own process (puts hand out, palm upper most, and shakes her head).

Sonia

The term 'just left hanging' was used by one of the respondents to describe what it was like to have no information for a period of time as to the outcome for the woman she believed that she should have delivered. In three accounts there is a pervading sense of the midwives experiencing a loss of professional control. It is possible that such a loss may have helped to fuel their intense feelings of irritation at not being able to bring closure to the stillbirth event and their part in it.

I don't know what happened to that girl because I was on night duty and I just went away, and obviously . . . sort of logistics of things, of dealing with the stillbirth, wasn't really dealt with there was no follow through for me. It was for me unsatisfactory . . . I was just left hanging (shakes her head).

Sally

I hate it when you go off and leave things unfinished . . . I didn't see her baby but I rang up that evening to see what she'd had and actually the midwife who was then looking after her recognised that I wanted to know what the baby was and how much it weighed . . . I would just hate, hate just to go off on holiday and never know what had happened to her . . . I was so worn out that weekend but I knew that I just had to see her in her home.

Claire

Now I was going on holiday the next day; this was going to be my last shift, for three weeks and really it was quite unfortunate in one respect. It felt like I was being taken out of the situation halfway through and I really needed to see it to the end.

Andrea

The ability to achieve closure for some of the midwives was seen as being sabotaged by memories of professional conflict.

YEARS DOWN THE LINE AND STILL STUCK WITH IT: PROFESSIONAL CONFLICT SURROUNDING A STILLBIRTH

Anger and conflict are common enough, but the anger and conflict felt around a death is marked by a context of irritability and bitterness (Parkes 1996). The frequent expression of personal anger, feelings of loneliness and insecurity can, as Parkes, identifies, result in the bereaved becoming socially isolated. Isolation can also stem from the perception that others have violated one's personal beliefs and moral values. The individual's philosophy of midwifery practice and what it means to be a midwife was, therefore, interlinked with how they saw the provision of midwifery and obstetric care at the time of the stillbirth.

It was particularly hard for the midwives to cope and move on from a stillbirth where the behaviour of colleagues clashed with the midwife's personal and professional belief systems, especially with regard to their relationship with the mother. In such emotional times, seeking someone to blame for loss is common.

Within this study, recrimination and attributing blame with associated feelings of anger and bitterness was not only seen by those midwives shouldering self-blame and guilt (see Chapter 7), but a few midwives also sought to blame others. Three midwives directed anger and blame at the loss of infant life on to another midwife or doctor. All three cited personal grievances regarding managerial decisions from a midwifery supervision perspective, the main one being that supervisors failed to identify or listen to the midwives' feelings of insecurity and left them professionally unprotected.

There is a sense that grief reactions appeared more intense and remained over a longer period of time if the stillbirths were categorised as senseless or preventable deaths.

Bereavement theorists agree that successful completion of mourning cannot be delineated in terms of time, but research has identified that the majority of people will find a comfortable psychological position, or degree of acceptance, within two years of the death (Worden 2003; Parkes 1996). There appeared to be little personal or professional closure on the stillbirths experienced by these three midwives, one that had occured 5 years previously and two 20 years previously, as they were seen as avoidable tragedies. Anger, conflict and alienation from professional colleagues remained largely unresolved.

Sally continued to bear feelings of 'justifiable' and intense anger towards two of her senior midwifery colleagues, one of whom she considered was culpable for a stillbirth that had occurred 20 years earlier. This caused her to see herself as 'a victim', for she argued that it was she, and not her two senior colleagues, who had been required to deliver the woman of her fresh stillbirth, complete the statutory documentation, prepare the baby for viewing and console the parents. Reflection and rationalisation emerged, but Sally could not justify the actions of her senior manager and supervisor of midwives at that time, for in her view the supervisor failed the mother and herself by not reviewing her colleague's professional practice. Her relationship with that supervisor of midwives became extremely strained. Sally's verbal and non-verbal communication were completely congruent, expressing how she was 'stuck with it . . . never been able to put the trauma to bed' and there was an accompanying feeling of anger, restlessness, frustration and impotence within her tone of voice.

> *I've always been angry about it and . . . I have never, never been able to resolve it . . . the managers did nothing . . . This was totally due to my colleague's misdemeanour, and that from my position has never been dealt with . . . I got the job of delivering, washing and presenting this dead baby . . . I got the whole lot!* (Heavy emphasis on the words and face alters, and right hand is put into a fist shape.)
>
> Sally

There is a repetition of the phrase 'stuck with it' in an account of another stillbirth by the same midwife. She continued to harbour deep resentment and had never found the opportunity to obtain closure; though she, like many of her colleagues in this study, had changed elements of her practice to incorporate learning from her experience. Many years later Sally became a supervisor of midwives. She spoke of encouraging junior colleagues to feel free to open up and discuss events and to reflect on their own behaviour and that of their colleagues. Sally's non-verbal actions as well as her words clearly identified that, even in adversity, personal reflection can promote professional learning; but consigning the event to supervisory history did not help her to feel comfortable with the memory.

> *Angry, yes I am, cos . . . I'm stuck with it . . . from a point of supervision they should have moved in big style but they didn't. You know, had it happened in this day and age, things would have been handled differently, where I work now as a midwifery supervisor, we have 'mumsy sessions'. I encourage staff to get stuff of their chest . . . and learn from events, but me I'm stuck with it* (bangs her hand down on her lap).
>
> Sally

In the following narratives the midwives expressed their anger because they felt that colleagues failed them and the family. Sophie and her client had no awareness that this pregnancy could only end in a stillbirth. That information should have been available several weeks before the birth, but it was misfiled. The end result would not have been any different, but Sophie considered that the process surrounding the child's birth could have been far less traumatic for both her client and herself but for this avoidable administrative mistake. The focus on the psychological outcome of the event, and her consistent use of the word 'we' confirms that she is referring to herself as well as the mother. She believes that a stillborn baby can be delivered in an atmosphere that welcomes its birth and acknowledges its death in a manner acceptable to the mother and to her as the known midwife. As Parkes (1996) hypothesises from his observations in hospices, when individuals, including staff, are given the right circumstances, they are able to discuss the impending death of another and often they are able to share some of the anticipatory grief, which each needs to feel. Thus, the shock of sudden unexpected death is prevented, with all its potential for blame, and the pain of loss can be anticipated and, to some extent, shared.

> *It upsets me greatly . . . I am very angry . . . because I think we could have had a psychologically much better outcome. For, had we known that the baby had congenital anomalies and would be stillborn, we could have had an open and frank discussion as to how the woman wanted to conduct her confinement and we'd have been ready for a birth and a death . . . the evidence had been there for weeks . . . hidden away . . .* (long pause) *it hung over me for a long time.*
>
> Sophie

Andrea valued consistency in medical or midwifery decision-making. She still carried anger towards a medical colleague who, five years previously, she considered acted out of professional character and thus created an avoidable tragedy. Her anger did not stop at him, for she turned it on herself and she claimed herself to be a perpetrator of harm to her client.

> *He* (the doctor) *totally disbelieved what we were seeing on the tracing . . . I couldn't believe it, we had never had any problems before with him . . . we argued again and again . . . I was so upset . . . he did not relay my concern to the consultant. I was so frustrated . . . I had tried to be professional and polite all the time . . . we lost that baby . . . and I blame myself as well as him . . . even though I had had numerous talks with the consultant over that lady . . . I am still carrying this five years on.*
>
> Andrea

These three midwives felt that in these instances they and their clients had lost personal control of the situations as well as losing their babies. This loss was very painful to them; they felt colleagues had failed them and their clients, and as such a professional apology was required.

PLACING BLAME AND THE NEED FOR APOLOGY

Weinberg (1995) explores how examining self-blame, seeking ways to make amends or apologising are ways of helping recovery from bereavement. This was significant when the midwives considered that they deserved a professional apology.

Lack of such apologies served to deepen their feelings and isolate them from the colleagues concerned. Weinberg stresses the importance of an individual's beliefs about responsibility and orderly control in their world when considering a death. Three midwives felt that midwifery supervision had let them down by not reviewing the practice of others and even falsely accusing them of professional incompetence. Only a professional and public apology could negate the deep feelings of hurt harboured by these midwives. Yet these three midwives did not have a midwifery supervision framework at that time that incorporated professional counselling alongside guided reflection. Had such a framework been in place, their feelings could have been acknowledged and support provided that would not only have enabled them to find an enduring place for their loss, but also helped them to regain their self-esteem and professional integrity.

> *Clinical supervision could have helped me to regain my self-control and professional integrity; in the end it alienated them both. I only got them back years later and then I was able to gain resolution to that event.*
>
> Sophie

Similar pleas for consideration of personal as well as professional accountability arose in further accounts. The midwives reported that working relationships became fraught when it was perceived that blame apportioning might ensue and professional and personal apprehension rapidly developed into deep defensiveness.

> *My supervisor said there is no provision for staff in the NHS to gain counselling . . . they said they were only interested in seeing my notes. I took a copy of everything . . . cos things changed and I felt like I was going into battle . . . I felt like the doctors were trying to lay the blame on me . . . I felt awful for it seemed . . . them and us, a sense of let's look after ourselves.*

Andrea

> *I was suspended and re-informed that I was an incompetent practitioner. All the questions were made of me, none about the doctor's practice! I heard nothing after that from the managers . . . But . . . I was exonerated totally . . . then I felt hostile and reluctant to go back to work. When I did, I was given a wide berth, and so I would not speak to them . . . I felt isolated. I never forgave them and I carried it as a huge burden for many years.*

Sophie

Sophie had insight into her own needs following that stillbirth: to have a grounded and secure sense of being accepted both as an individual and as a midwife.

> *I needed to go back to work, to touch base and feel safe and secure about me and my professional practice. I needed them not to have judged me before the outcome of the investigation. I needed one of them to say, 'you are ok as a person' . . . to have faith. After everything came out, no one offered me anything . . . no reversal of their judgement made of me.*

Sophie

Midwifery supervision, at that time, lacked such insight and left Sally with 'nowhere to go' with the intense feelings of anger that she held around other colleagues.

> *I still feel that anger towards them today . . . no one said anything to that midwife . . . nowhere to go with any emotional feelings . . . the profession, supervision, did it let me down? Yes there was nowhere to go . . . the incident, though clear in my mind, I don't recall how I dealt with it . . . 20 years and the pain is still in there . . . no one said 'sorry'.*

Sally

The accounts of these three midwives are full of this sense of 'nowhere to go, no one said sorry'. One is left with the vision of them desperately seeking some place to deposit their anger and frustration at colleagues. Despite this, Sally considered that, for future midwives faced with tragic events, things have changed and can continue to change for the better through the introduction of reflective practice.

It is quite regular now to see midwives waiting to talk to their supervisor in the morning following a night shift. To say 'oh I just wanted to talk about the way I have handled something' . . . mumsy time is very, very important.

Sally

Sally's past experiences of midwifery supervision were balanced, to a degree, by an appreciation that this statutory regulation of midwives is changing positively and can now be practised in an atmosphere of anticipatory support. Her words and those of Andrea and Sophie emphasise the importance of midwives not only understanding but being seen to acknowledge a fellow midwife's feelings around loss. This acceptance, together with offering a chance to talk about the situation and her feelings, is inextricably linked to a midwife's perception of being supported, even to the extent of requesting an apology. Such support is crucial: it is a profoundly enabling gesture that allows the midwife to find the means of achieving closure.

NEW BABIES COME ALONG

The delivery of a healthy baby is the joy of being a midwife. This is only surpassed by feelings of pleasure when the mother, who has suffered a stillbirth in the past, gives birth to a live healthy baby, supported by her known midwife.

Several midwives described trying to ensure that they were informed of births to mothers with a previous history of stillbirth. Many women are pregnant again within a few months of a stillbirth (Boyle 1997) and the midwives were aware of this and sought to maintain knowledge of their childbearing. Five of the twelve midwives made direct reference to their feelings at receiving news that new babies had been born to these women, with whom they had a tragic connection. In the opinion of four out of the five midwives, knowing that new babies are anticipated served to aid them in finding closure on the previous stillbirth.

I cannot remember how long after that happened that she came back in with a full-term pregnancy . . . but she did say 'thank you' and 'you did all that you could back then'.

Susanna

When the time came to book them again with a new pregnancy they both came together and they both agreed to see me, it made such a difference.

Lesley

Andrea inferred that her channels of communication with her colleagues were primed to inform her when a woman whom she had delivered of a stillbirth became pregnant again. She, like Linda, expressed an important need to know. Their accounts convey unspoken evidence of their relief as well as joy that a new baby was shortly to be born. However, these two accounts bear witness to concerns that both midwives harboured for the women with whom they had a connection.

It was two years later, no it wasn't (head goes back and she looks up at the ceiling, eyes moving from side to side). *No, no it would be one year later to the day that I saw her in the fetal assessment clinic, being monitored again and about 36 weeks pregnant. I knew she was pregnant again, one of the other community midwives had told me . . . I felt so happy for her, but it all seemed so soon and I wondered if she had recovered emotionally.*

Andrea

She's had another baby since and I am so pleased about that . . . cos I thought she probably wouldn't. I thought that having to have a termination and then a perinatal death that she'd never get pregnant again, but she did and I feel so positive for her. My colleagues said to me, 'it's lovely to see you smiling again' (gives a large and relaxed smile, her hands are held limply on her knees).

Linda

The statement by Linda that her colleagues were happy to see her smiling again serves to illustrate how she had been in a state of professional grief after the stillbirth. Her body language was relaxed, her smile appeared genuine.

In stark contrast, the arrival of a new baby only brought partial resolution to one midwife. A previous client informed Sophie that the mother with whom she had a tragic link had given birth again. While outwardly expressing happiness for the newly delivered mother, Sophie acknowledged that she did not find the solace she craved in that news.

The resolution of part of my burden, if you like, came recently, when the lady had another baby, and requested of her community midwife, why she wasn't seeing me . . . and asked to visit me which I did and there she was with a new baby, and very pleased to see me . . . she said to me 'I'm ok I'm fine' . . . but I wasn't.

Sophie

Sophie knew that this mother held her in high esteem, despite the tragedy that befell her first pregnancy, and she hoped that Sophie would visit her in the future. When the interview ended, Sophie sat for a long while and then very quietly explained that she had lost more than a baby. She spoke of the loss of her professional integrity and confidence. Several other midwives spoke of their feelings of grief that were bound up with loss of some aspect of professional integrity. Seeking resolution to this loss proved to be as painful and perhaps even more difficult for the midwives concerned than the loss of the babies, for it involved professional conflict.

Most of the midwives interviewed felt that they needed to talk of the reasons why the stillbirth events impacted on them in such a way as to cause emotional and physical distress. These midwives described how they classified their midwifery and medical colleagues into those who may help them by listening and offering support to articulate and release pent-up anxieties and the others whose actions or remarks served only to psychologically impede any disclosure.

Meeting with the mothers at an appropriate time after the stillbirth to re-establish a connection and allow discussion was important to these midwives. Such a meeting allowed the midwife to discuss her part in the event, her professional actions, and words; and for some midwives it is clear that this was their most acceptable means of obtaining closure. This was especially helpful for the midwife when the woman thanked her, or spoke warmly of the care the midwife had given her around the stillbirth. The ultimate tribute to that professional care was when the mother requested her care again in the next pregnancy, though the fragmented way in which NHS midwifery care is organised made this difficult even when the mother wished it.

In retrospect, we feel that 'closure' may not have been an appropriate word for midwives with regard to stillbirth (Klass, Silverman and Nickman 1996). We ourselves have learned that one does not bring to closure such profound experiences; one learns instead to reshape them as experiences that contribute to personal growth and development and store them elsewhere in one's memories. Experiences around stillbirth and the emotions generated do not suddenly disappear but merely fade into a state of acceptance.

It is important to acknowledge that while some of these 12 midwives may have reached a level of acceptance around the stillbirth events they chose to narrate, entering into a study such as this provided a catalyst that decisively awakened those painful memories. It appeared significant to 11 of the respondents that they keep the typed transcripts of their own narratives and most of the midwives stated that rereading the transcripts helped them rationalise aspects of those stillbirth events. Resolution is clearly a continuing process.

CHAPTER 9

Independent midwives' responses to stillbirths and neonatal deaths

Fifteen IMs were interviewed concerning nine stillbirths and six neonatal deaths. They have not been given pseudonyms for reasons of confidentiality (*see* Chapter 1). These midwives were self-employed and contracted to provide continuity of care to their clients and therefore knew them well.

The women had booked with IMs because they wanted continuity of care and in many cases because they wished to make decisions about their care, which would not have been available to them within the NHS. For instance, most of the women wanted home births but various risk factors would have made this choice unavailable to them within the NHS. Thus, these IMs had been more closely involved with their clients and their individual decision-making than is usual in the NHS.

In 10 of the 15 cases, the parents did not consent to post-mortem examinations. This limits the extent to which it is possible to ascertain cause of death and created considerable uncertainty with which the parents and their midwives had to cope.

In seven cases, all the professionals involved with the case agreed that no other management in labour could have saved the baby who died. This knowledge provided important justification and comfort to the midwives concerned. In some cases, the midwives felt that an elective caesarean may have saved the baby but the mother had declined this option and the midwives respected her choice. In other cases, the midwives felt that better inter-professional communication by NHS staff, especially following transfer to hospital, may have saved the baby.

The self-employed status of these midwives carried considerable potential for isolation and blame from NHS colleagues. It also gave them the autonomy to provide care in partnership with the mother and to build their own support networks.

THE CONSOLATION OF GIVING THE BEST POSSIBLE CARE

A good labour

For those women who did not have caesarean sections, the IMs endeavoured to ensure that they laboured as they had originally planned.

In one case, where the woman transferred to hospital in labour because there was no fetal heartbeat, the IM insisted on the woman having access to a pool and she had 'The best birth she ever had, a lovely water birth'. Another, whose baby died before labour, 'had a very, very sensitive birth and met her baby in a dignified way, which she wanted'. Such care was a comfort to the bereaved mother and the midwife.

Postnatal support

Immediate postnatal care was very important to the IMs and they worked hard to create positive memories for families in tragic circumstances. They respected and supported the families, and appreciation of that support from parents or other professionals was a comfort to them.

> *She* (the supervisor of midwives) *said, 'If you're going to lose your baby, this is as good as it gets'. . . . When she walked into the room . . . the baby was on a sheepskin in the middle of the room with the children kneeling round her, feeling her hands and looking at her . . . They kept the baby in the house until about midnight and then decided that she was deteriorating and then they decided, having thought they'd keep her overnight, that they would actually call the undertaker . . . they look back on that time and we did amazing hand and feet prints with the children's poster paints and it was all slightly surreal. And made some supper – because the children needed to eat and so we were all sitting at the table with X with her baby over her shoulder. Holding on . . . they are committed Christians and . . . they just had this sense that death is part of life.*
>
> (stillbirth at home)

Where there was no transfer to hospital, the IMs gave a great deal of immediate care, liaising with other professionals including funeral directors, GPs, the police and the coroner. As in the pregnancy, the midwives worked with great flexibility to support the mothers' choices and to facilitate their decision-making when the parents did not know the options available to them.

> *We sat with the mother, we sat with the twins, we took lots of pictures. We took the baby when she was ready. And, having spoken to her afterwards, she said that, had she been in hospital she feels that it would have become a very, very different experience . . . People would have been rushing in and rushing out. The baby would have been taken away from her and she just feels that, when she was ready, we took the baby to the chapel of rest, not a stranger. I held him in the car and it really gave her a lot of comfort. It was quite difficult to hold the baby because I could feel his deterioration on the journey, even to the chapel of rest. But, out of respect for her, we*

did that. And so that left me certainly with a feeling that we had concluded life's cycle too.

(stillborn, macerated, second twin, born at home, no admission to hospital)

In most of these cases the postnatal care given by the IM was extended and highly supportive in practical and emotional terms.

I did go and sit with them both. There was a lot of intensive work around [grief], in the immediate postnatal period I was there a lot. And I did go back to sit and talk through with them some issues that they had . . . [later].

In a number of cases, the postnatal support included the wider family.

We did a huge amount of talking about things postnatally with both the parents, both sets of grandparents and her sister. We spent a long, long time talking things through with them.

In most cases the IMs attended the funeral, sometimes travelling considerable distances to do so.

The midwives acted as the mother's advocate in many respects.

I went to the coroner's hearing. I didn't have to give evidence but I went with the grandparents, the parents couldn't face it . . . It was a woman coroner. She was wonderful and it was really good because the grandparents were able to hear the findings.

We sought legal advice from a trusted, very woman-centred barrister . . . and she said they need to write a letter saying they want . . . to reserve the right for a second autopsy . . . and that changed everything. It changed the sense of justice and control for the family . . . and I suspect it changed the pathologist's attitude.

In one case this advocacy extended to making a formal complaint to the Independent Police Complaints Commission on behalf of the family concerning the behaviour of the police after the baby's death. This lengthy process ended in the parents receiving an apology and the reassurance that a specialist team now deals with unexpected infant deaths in that area. That reassurance was a consolation to the midwife and to the parents. The knowledge this IM gained in the course of this case was shared with other IMs in similar circumstances later.

Most of the mothers were very appreciative of their IM's care and cards and other signs of that appreciation were treasured by the midwives.

She wrote us a really beautiful poem, a beautiful, beautiful poem about her two babies and about our care.

(stillborn, second twin at home)

In all but one of these cases postnatal care was given by the IM and they described it as hard but therapeutic for themselves as well as for the parents. The process of giving the best postnatal care they could was important in the resolution of the midwives' grief.

The one case where the parents declined IM care and received postnatal care from NHS community midwives was very traumatic for the IM concerned. She said that she had learned from the case that it was very important to maintain a postnatal relationship with the family.

> *Keep close to a family that is bereaved or damaged or traumatised, try and keep close to them. For yourself and for them. . . . This case is so awful because I haven't been able to resolve things for me adequately and the family haven't either. And now I think that the time is too far gone, I don't think we can.*

This case shows how the IMs saw the resolution of their grief as interwoven with the resolution of the grief of the bereaved family and how resolution could be helped by giving care that they saw as truly 'with woman'. Where this was not possible the midwife suffered a loss, not only from the death, but also from not being able to use her professional skills.

Subsequent pregnancies

Though the subsequent reproductive history of some of the women is not known, the continuity of care and connection is remarkable. In 5 of the 15 cases the woman booked with the same IM in her next pregnancy. In 4 other cases the woman booked an elective caesarean in her next pregnancy and in one of these cases the woman talked through her options with the IM before booking with a consultant. 'She did consider coming with me and in the end didn't', after weighing all the options in discussion with her IM. In another of these cases the woman also booked her IM to give her support as a doula.

Some mothers kept in touch with their IMs, though they decided to have different care in the next pregnancy. One, who had left the area, booked an elective caesarean at 38 weeks in her next pregnancy and wrote to the IM after the birth; they are still in touch.

Where the relationship continued, the midwifery support concerning the bereavement also continued.

> (The next baby delivered by the same midwife) *was another little boy and they knew it was another little boy and it was the little girl that they had lost. And so we had a lot of work to do through that – that she, she feels cheated at not having a daughter, and I've got daughters – you know, there's a lot there still. But we still talk. She still rings me up every now and then.*

Another IM adds, on her Christmas cards to the family, 'remembering X [name of dead baby]' and the mother has told her that this continuing acknowledgement of the child they lost as part of their family is important to them.

All the IMs felt that postnatal care was very important, particularly after the death of a baby. For a considerable number of the mothers, their relationship with the IM and the trust they felt in her lasted a long time.

The potential for reciprocal resolution of grief within the midwife–mother relationship was very striking in these interviews and the midwives saw this as important for all concerned. They also valued the way in which this mutual resolution could extend over prolonged periods of time. This was only possible because they had control of their practice as IMs in ways that were not possible for their NHS colleagues. In this situation their clients also exercised far greater autonomy than NHS patients.

MATERNAL AUTONOMY

The way in which the IMs worked with the women differed from the way the NHS would have worked with them, where the women would have booked for a standard package of care.

Supporting women who took responsibility for their pregnancies was fundamental to the IMs' philosophy of care. Some felt this was essential.

> Interviewer: *Did you feel she took responsibility for her pregnancy and its outcomes?*
> IM: *Yes, very much or I wouldn't have worked with her.*

This level of maternal responsibility was demonstrated in these cases where women made decisions that would not have been available to them within the NHS. It also had considerable implications in terms of both guilt and control where death occurred.

The IM care was not standardised and was very respectful of the women's choices and preferences. This was demonstrated in major issues, such as booking women for home birth that had been refused an NHS home booking. Sometimes this was demonstrated by the IM going to great lengths to arrange a hospital booking that fitted the woman's needs.

> *I felt that I totally supported her . . . She went the medical route the first time and ended up with an outcome that she didn't – that was awful* (a severely handicapped baby) *and this time she went the midwifery route, tried to do things differently . . . I've never worked so hard before or after to negotiate things within an NHS hospital. I worked really, really hard to . . . cover all bases. And we end up with a dead baby. But I think she did take responsibility.*
> (twin pregnancy, planned vaginal birth after previous caesarean,
> in hospital with two IMs)

The IMs' continuing respect for the women's autonomy and their choices allowed for much more variation in care than would have been possible within the NHS.

> *We talked a lot about monitoring in labour . . . She had a need for privacy and a need to be interfered with as little as possible and she wanted to keep things as low key as*

we possibly could. So . . . the plan was just listen in intermittently to the babies and be free to mobilise . . . We talked a lot about continuous fetal monitoring; she didn't feel that would be of benefit.

(twin pregnancy, planned vaginal birth after caesarean [VBAC])

The autonomy of the mother and the midwife, within an ongoing relationship, which both had chosen, created a degree of reciprocity that was supportive for both. The IMs' comfort zones were, therefore, much wider than those of their NHS colleagues.

Our comfort zone is huge . . . Give women more leeway and the trust works two ways and they take your advice.

They also saw this as enabling a trusting relationship, which could make care safer.

We, the IMs, are all about choice, giving these high-risk women a loving comfort zone for them to birth the way they know they can and a loving supportive relationship with their own midwife. With time to foster this relationship then trust builds up and in the event of suspected deviations then the woman will trust her IM's judgement and transfer in for appropriate care in hospital.

The IMs took pride in meeting the women's needs.

She was challenging [to the community midwives with whom she originally booked], not having scans and she declined all screening (i.e. ultrasound scans [USS] and bloods). *She was very nervous of even having her blood pressure taken.*

The IM spent a lot of time supporting this woman and building up her confidence.

Nevertheless, some women stretched the IMs' comfort zones. In one case, the midwife observed she 'would have wanted to monitor her more in labour', but accepted that 'she was resistant to the amount of surveillance' the midwife would have chosen. One woman did not call the IM to her labour; the IM went anyway because the woman had informed her that her membranes had ruptured but she did not want the IM to attend her then. The IMs did not stereotype or blame these women.

CHOICES AND ALLIES

Since these women had made choices that were not acceptable within the NHS, there were times when the IMs felt they were the woman's only ally. The IMs felt it was particularly important to take that role where, without an IM, the woman would have delivered unattended.

Half of me feels that if I'd turned into a different sort of person and bullied her into hospital, then that might have been the right thing to do as per keeping the baby alive.

However, the other side of me was – I was the only person on her side . . . because another thing she said to me during the postnatal period was, 'I did it, didn't I? I gave birth to my baby. I can do it.' And so another part of me was like, if I had bullied her into hospital and the baby died anyway, who would she have had on her side?

(VBAC breech who felt she was 'bullied into a caesarean with her previous breech')

The second midwife in the above case also reflected on the possibility that if her colleague had 'bullied' the woman to get her to transfer to hospital, she may have 'ordered you out of the house . . . so you risked betraying her at the time she needed you most'. In another case, the midwife reflected:

I know there are midwives who would have gone out to her and transferred in possibly earlier than I did. I don't know whether they would have done that out of fear or out of knowledge, but I have been at some very challenging births that have had really positive outcomes at home. And I don't feel I made the wrong decisions as a midwife. And the woman did not want to go to hospital and I was the one saying 'I'm calling an ambulance now'. And if she had objected, I wouldn't have done because that would have been her right to do that, but I felt at that point she needed me to be really clear . . . What is really hard to balance is the women who are so frightened of NHS care or going into hospital that they put themselves into really complex situations based on fear. And that is the hardest thing, I think, about independent midwifery where you support women in their choices not where you goad them into doing what you want them to do.

The IMs' efforts to maintain this balance impacted on their relationships with NHS colleagues.

BLAME AND ALLIANCES

The choices made by the mothers in this study together with their midwives' respect for their clients' decisions could create tensions for the IMs in their relationships with NHS colleagues.

One woman was told by a consultant during her pregnancy that she had to have an elective caesarean. The consultant told the IM, 'we can always get women to do what we want them to do' and she clearly expected the IM to do the same. This consultation did not make the woman agree to an elective caesarean; rather it strengthened her resolve to labour.

In the investigations that followed another case, the IM reported being told that she 'listens to women too much' by both a supervisor of midwives and the Nursing and Midwifery Council.

On a few occasions, the IM felt that NHS staff blamed her for the death.

[T]he consultant was trying to blame me. She verbally said it to me and I debated it with her . . . I was very clear about it and I was not budging and I was not going to

be bullied into taking responsibility for this . . . I think that's the hardest thing cos the bullying is so extensive.

(planned VBAC, caesarean section of stillborn baby revealed torn broad liga-
ment – 1 hour and 40 minutes after admission to hospital)

The IM just quoted also felt that the mother was 'put under a lot of pressure to have a PM [post-mortem], which she declined.

In some cases, the midwives felt that NHS closed ranks against them.

When we arrived with the baby – straight into special care they just, the staff were just horrible. It was like a wall went up.

The IMs felt that, in some cases, NHS staff blamed the mother for her baby's death. In one case they 'threatened to report her to social services as an unfit mother', but this threat was not carried out.

Blaming and lack of collegial behaviour from NHS staff could make IMs feel powerless and victimised.

[The NHS] takes all the power away and takes all the responsibility away except when they want to shove it back at you. When they are ready to shove it back at you they will. Yeah.

Blaming could produce guilt, for mothers and midwives.

[H]ad this been handled differently then we would all be much more settled about it . . . It reminds me – I read this quote from Atonement, *Ian McEwan's book – it's the beginning of one of the chapters and it's so beautiful. It's how guilt redefined the methods of self-torture, threading the beads of detail, into an eternal loop, a rosary to be fingered for a lifetime. And that resonates because there are aspects of what happened with this case that are going to remain and are never going to be put away properly because we've never had the opportunity to do so.*

This was the one case where the IM did not have contact with the mother after the birth. In most of the cases, midwives and mothers did not experience blaming and manipulation, but where they did the effect was devastating.

Maternal self-blame and blaming by the family

The IMs were very aware of the devastating effects of the loss of a child upon a family. They were also aware of mothers' doubts about their own decisions.

I do vividly recall this woman saying to me 'What have I done?' when I waited at home with her to complete the labour process while her baby had gone to hospital.

The IMs endeavoured to provide support around these doubts, often by sharing them.

> *I think there was that feeling that perhaps there was that lack of caution or perhaps she felt I should have pushed her in [to hospital]. There was, there was that doubt. But we've talked about it and we can both acknowledge we can never take it away, that doubt, because it's in my head too.*

As well as the potential for self-blame after such a loss, the IMs discussed the potential for the mother to be blamed by some family members.

> *I think it was really important that we all worked so hard with the extended family . . . The dad's parents took it worst and they almost blamed the mum and she was obviously blaming herself.*

Postnatal support was extended to those members of the family who felt this was appropriate for them.

The midwives reflected on these cases and discussed them with colleagues and with the families concerned.

> *It took a huge amount of work for us all* (the family and both IMs) *to come to terms with the fact that if she had gone in and had the section at 38, 39 weeks . . . or even if she'd gone in when she went into labour, if she'd gone in the night before. And it was very much her decision that she would stay at home. X* (the other IM) *and I, . . . talked about it and felt that we would have been happier if she had gone in . . . She felt she wanted to have a rest . . . she wasn't aggressively against our advice, had we been stronger with our advice she might well have gone in. I mean if we'd bullied her and harassed, or come across stronger . . . She didn't book me to bully her . . . she booked [me] . . . to get out of being bullied.*

Some of the 'huge amount of work' is done as part of postnatal care with the parents and family, as mentioned previously. Where that is not possible, this is very hard for the midwife.

> *I still feel desperately sad for the family. My family and [others] feel very angry at the couple. I can't get past feeling anything but sadness for the couple, rightly or wrongly. I do feel frustrated at times with them and I feel a bit angry that they never gave us the opportunity to meet. We've never met with them, never had the opportunity to finish that off. And it's too late now. I have no wish now to meet with them.*

SUPERVISORY SUPPORT

There were many cases of excellent support from supervisors of midwives and this support was greatly appreciated. This may reflect the changes in supervision between 2002, when the data in previous chapters were collected, and 2009 when this study was conducted. Some issues remained the same.

Two cases were referred to the Local Supervisory Authority (LSA) and the LSA

Midwifery Officer (LSAMO) conducted supervisory investigations into the deaths. These investigations had a further, prolonged impact upon the midwives.

> IM: *Very, very scared, about what would happen to me. Very scared for however long it took for the investigation . . . over a year . . . beating myself up that someone would say I killed the baby.*
> Interviewer: *What was the outcome of that?*
> IM: *No case to answer.*
> (stillbirth at home, mother refused to transfer to hospital in labour)

Supervisory reviews could be lengthy. Some IMs suffered greatly in this process, against which they had no appeal.

> *I feel very hard done by, by my profession. I feel badly let down by supervision and very, very angry at the LSAMO who has . . . I think behaved badly. And part of the pain that the parents have been left in I think is largely due to the handling of the situation early on. And I think it was badly handled and I find it difficult to forgive because . . . if she'd handled it differently the parents would have been better. I have had to have psychotherapy and ongoing counselling as well. So it hasn't been an easy three-and-a-half years . . .*

In one case, issues arising from the review went on for four years, although the midwives were exonerated.

MUTUAL SUPPORT FROM COLLEAGUES

There were many cases of excellent support from NHS staff, which was greatly appreciated. All the midwives received vital support from other IMs. Sometimes this was an immediate IM colleague.

> *We cried. We cried an awful lot that morning . . . and we were also very numb.*
> (two IMs after leaving the parents)

Where there were two IMs they supported each other through their experience of loss.

> *When you are supporting parents as much as you should be supporting parents then you put your own grief to the back and it wasn't until sometime later that – yeah I can remember sitting in the car saying to [the second midwife] 'I don't feel as if I've cried for that baby'. And you need to do that.*

This IM described her colleague as 'an absolute rock'. The situation was harder when there was only one IM present at the labour, which was usually the case with singleton pregnancies.

> *I said 'I'll give you all the support I can and you need to talk to our colleague and you need to talk to the bereavement midwife. And if you want to call me at any time, just call me at any time. But right this minute I need to deal with it. I'm devastated myself'.*

The nature of the IMs' lives, constantly on call, meant that the loss also had an impact on their families.

> *[I]t's not an easy process. Turned our family upside down. I had my . . . [child], in the car when I got the call [from the parent] saying the baby's not breathing. I'm trying to find an ambulance and being put on hold. A baby's death is very stressful and it has a big impact on our own families. I've lost a baby myself; I know what it's like. But again, I thought, that's why I'm meant to be the midwife for this family because I do know what it's like. It's horrible . . . That's just one of the tough things of the job. And I guess it never gets any easier.*
>
> (neonatal death)

All the IMs interviewed spoke of the reciprocal support network of other IMs who they could 'ring up at 2 a.m. if I need to talk'. There was a lot of discussion amongst the IMs and a lot of sharing of information. Knowledge that one IM gained as a result of supporting parents after a stillbirth was available to other IMs and this was referred to in several interviews as practically helpful and making the midwife feel less isolated.

The midwives thought a lot about these cases.

> *And when you're working independently I think you're automatically a midwife who goes back over something – everything that you do and say. And obviously it knocks your confidence, I mean nobody likes handing a dead baby to a mother.*

Sometimes the very unexpectedness of the baby's death took its toll on the midwife, despite excellent support.

> *This was so much out of the blue and the other ones* (deaths) *you've seen stuff leading up to it or – and I just don't think they get any easier. And I, I had loads of support from the bereavement midwife, I had loads of support from the obstetrician, the neonatologist, cos they understood I was quite distressed and so they made time for me . . . But this was so unexplained that I just thought, 'I don't know if I want to do this anymore' . . . I just saw out my caseload. I didn't take on anybody else . . . I just saw out who I had to see.*
>
> (cot death)

Two IMs ceased to practice as a result of these deaths. In the case quoted above (cot death) the mother and midwife received support from all the NHS staff involved; in the other case both the IMs involved felt they were bullied by NHS staff. One IM partnership split up as a result of another case, in which the family blamed the IMs for the death.

THE PHILOSOPHY OF INDEPENDENT MIDWIFERY

These midwives and most of their clients were able to tolerate a greater degree of uncertainty and paradox than is usual in the NHS.

> *Death is so much part of life; I think as we get older we realise that. And the tragedies of babies dying – babies do die and sometimes mothers die and sometimes there's no one to blame. You know, the Americans have a very good phrase: shit happens. And it does happen and sometimes, yes, we could have done things better but who's to know that the outcome would have been different or not. Things I have said to you, my opinion, I believe. But I don't know and neither do the parents.*

The clinical notes and the interviews contained many words of wisdom. The value placed upon trusting, continuing relationships is very clear.

> *[T]he things that independent midwives gain often is the joy of that close relationship. But, when something sad like this happens, I think it's still a really beneficial relationship to have with a client. Because I think it meant that she has a wonderful, dignified memory of her beautiful baby . . . There's part of you thinks – well, maybe it would make me falter and think, I'm not doing this because it's given me such heartache and, yes, I cried and it's a very sad event. But it did make me think that part of the thing we can give to our clients is . . . that relationship of trust that can transcend all boundaries . . . that maybe hospital protocols would not allow.*

There were certainly examples of exemplary care and of IMs using their experience to benefit future clients, which was clearly important in the resolution of the midwife's own grief.

> *I think that the thing that can be learned from this case is that death is part of – part and parcel of the process we work with. And just sometimes it can be nice. That sounds a really stupid thing to say, nobody wants their baby to die, we all want a live healthy baby, but it doesn't have to be full of blame, full of who did what wrong. [In the NHS] you have to have an answer, everything has to fit into a box. It can be just part of what we do. And part of what we do is helping women grieve, accept that sometimes babies die without anybody to blame and anybody's fault and no matter what we do that's going to happen sometimes . . . that is something I learned on that case. And I talk about that to other clients, you know, when they ask me, 'Have you ever had a baby die?' And I say 'Yes. I have had a baby die and it wasn't all a negative thing.'*

In many ways these IMs' experiences of loss were similar to those of their NHS colleagues. They certainly grieved for the babies who died and unexpected deaths were particularly traumatic. As they were self-employed, there was no sense in which a stillbirth was allocated to them, or that their care was limited by the requirements of managers. They knew the mothers and families well in each case, so each death was one to which they felt a close connection. Like their NHS colleagues, they suffered particularly when other professional losses were added to that of the death: where they could not provide further care to the mother, where they were not allowed to practise until the case was investigated or where the death really shook their clinical confidence.

These IMs had the opportunities afforded them by continuity of care and they were free from the institutional constraints, which loom large in the working lives of their NHS colleagues. This enabled them to identify and empathise with the women in their care. (Their pattern of speech and use of pronouns was more inclusive than any I have heard in a long career of interviewing NHS staff.) These midwives found consolation and resolution of their own grief in giving care tailored to the individual needs of their clients. Their relationships with clients were in many ways reciprocal, as were their relationships with colleagues. Being self-employed could have left them isolated, especially when relationships with NHS staff in a case were not good; they also lacked the protection of being NHS employees. They therefore worked to create and maintain a strong mutual support network amongst IMs.

CHAPTER 10

Making sense of loss around stillbirth

COPING WITH LOSS AROUND STILLBIRTH

The death of a baby inevitably produces sadness in the midwife; beyond this sadness many stillbirths produced feelings of loss and grief, which could be profound. Marris (1996) sees grief as 'a reaction to the disintegration of the whole structure of meaning' dependent on a relationship (47). Thus, in stillbirth the midwife loses not just the infant life, which she mourns with the parents, but also the structure of meaning fundamental to her work in supporting mothers at the start of a new life. Stillbirth takes away a basic part of her professional reason for being.

Where the death was sudden and unexpected, the midwives interviewed also experienced shock, anger and disbelief that could have physical manifestations. These responses were closely linked with feelings of guilt and blame. These experiences of professional grief produced a degree of suffering beyond that of sadness and required more skill in its handling and integration into midwives' professional experience.

Other grief-inducing losses associated with stillbirths were largely determined by the context and associated professional meaning. These losses could include loss of relationships with the mother of the baby and with colleagues who sought to avoid the mother and the carer involved with the stillbirth. These relationship losses produced varying degrees of professional isolation for the midwife, which could be deeply felt. Other losses were linked with the midwife's professional identity. These ranged from self-doubt and self-blame with varying degrees of loss of professional self-esteem, to extreme cases where the midwife was suspended from her work while the death was investigated and she experienced loss of her practice and thereby her professional identity, as well as loss of all working relationships. These factors together produced profound feelings of helplessness and deep grief, which again linked with guilt and blame.

The memories of stillbirths stayed with midwives as images; sometimes of a family with their dead child, or a bonnet or the wiping away of a tear, and sometimes these images carried a terrifying implication of judgement. We have described them as stained glass windows because they are vivid, set and composed of separate, precisely remembered panes, which together can produce small single images or complex scenes of doom and judgement. Whatever the image they contain, windows carry a graphic message and they let in light. Light can clarify the image concerned or illuminate other possible responses.

Loss shocks us and disrupts the story of our lives and our professional practice, therefore efforts and strategies are required in order to cope.

IMMEDIATE COPING STRATEGIES

Organisational support could provide a framework for the practical tasks around stillbirth, especially where there were clear protocols and lists of tasks to be done and forms to be completed; but it was human support, often brief and at a very practical level, which was really experienced as helpful.

Midwives practising in hospitals spoke of avoidance strategies around stillbirth. They mainly described these strategies as exercised by other midwives, but they spoke with insight and understanding of midwives who avoided giving care to mothers with a known intrauterine death or who sought to distance themselves from relationship with the woman if they were required to give such care. They also spoke of midwives avoiding colleagues who were caring for women with known intrauterine deaths in case they were themselves drawn into that emotionally demanding care.

As our analyses progressed we came to realise that the midwives were not only avoiding the next stillbirth, but also were avoiding reopening previous experiences of stillbirth, which they had not come to terms with and that remained painful. Accumulation of unprocessed grief has a very negative effect upon the emotions, freezing our emotional responses and resulting in an inability to empathise and eventually an inability to function (Lamers 1997; Parkes 2002). This creates a situation where avoidance appears to be the only coping strategy.

Yet midwives described how they coped much better when helped by colleagues. This could be with unpleasant and unfamiliar tasks, such as tissue sampling, or colleagues checking that all the paperwork was complete, expressing empathy, offering a listening ear or taking over the care of the mother when the midwife sought a short period of respite. Midwives understood that colleagues distanced themselves for fear that they too would become embroiled in an emotionally highly charged experience. Yet this knowledge of their colleagues' coping strategies served only to reinforce some of the midwives' experiences of isolation.

Those midwives who considered that they were well supported during intense periods of professional care-giving appeared to fare better psychologically than those who felt alienated and abandoned. They also seemed less likely to resort to self-blame, though such findings can only be very tentative as our samples were small and our studies qualitative. Where support was offered, midwives felt they could request brief but refreshing periods of respite from the immediate care of the mother. The activity of removing oneself for short periods of emotional respite is rarely an unprofessional act; it is one of self-care. Few midwives felt able to ask for such help unless it was specifically offered, when it made a tremendous difference.

Feeling positively supported often followed an empathic colleague briefly validating their feelings and emphasising that they were not alone. Such actions could also transform the midwife's view of her helpful colleague and be seen as role modelling for her own future practise. Nevertheless, such behaviour was unusual and, in hospital, avoidance was a more common coping strategy.

Thus, there was a real tension between the two immediate coping strategies. Avoidance protected the midwife by taking her away from the threatening situation and also prevented the midwife in that situation from getting the support she needed to practice at her best. Avoidance, by definition, does not enable the midwife to develop her skills and therefore is self-reinforcing as a coping strategy.

Avoidance was only possible where care was fragmented and the death already diagnosed or suspected. Hospital midwives could not control the cases allocated to them. They saw the allocation of stillbirths as arbitrary, which provoked considerable anxiety. Several recalled the allocation of women with known intrauterine deaths to their care on labour ward as a brutal initiation into dealing with death: 'it's your turn now' – not a gently supported extension of their skills. Such experiences made midwives fearful and were likely to lead to future avoidance. The industrial model of care means that considerable numbers of stillbirths occur on labour wards, so the need for such avoidance can be experienced relatively frequently, thus reinforcing this coping strategy. The descriptions of labour wards had a frantic element to them and such frantic activity can inhibit learning and risk-taking and throw midwives back upon their defensive reactions.

The option of avoidance was not available where the death was unexpected, especially during labour. This experience shocked all concerned. This was made worse where colleagues avoided both the midwife and her client so that the midwife felt that all the care around the death was heaped on her and she was stuck with it.

Where there was continuity of carer, mainly in independent midwifery, avoidance was not possible, nor was it desired, as the midwife already had a relationship with the mother and a commitment to that family. These midwives offered continuing support to their clients. Their descriptions of their work around stillbirths were very calm, in sharp contrast to the descriptions of busy labour wards. They controlled their workload and encountered stillbirths relatively rarely.

Those who offered continuity of care, both IMs and community midwives, also offered and received the most colleague support. Colleague support around loss was described at length by IMs, whose work is defined by continuity of care, and they very consciously developed and cherished their mutual support networks.

LONGER-TERM STRATEGIES: MAKING SENSE OF GRIEF

There are clearly many ways of making sense of our experiences. How we go about this, and what is seen as sense, is determined, to a large extent, by what is felt to be possible in our social context. The role models available to us, our reading, our beliefs and our friends can all increase the options available to us in this regard.

Resolution

Much of the literature on grief and loss supposes that grief is resolved at some point, and the bonds with the deceased severed so that the bereaved person can 'let go' and 'move on' (Parkes 1998; Bowlby 1991). Few of the midwives we interviewed spoke of the resolution of grief. Writing of her own stillbirth, McCracken (2009) acknowledges that 'life goes on but that death goes on, too, that a person who is dead is a long, long, story' (13). Our own experiences of loss echo this observation and together with the experiences of the midwives interviewed, lead us to conclude that such grief may not be finally resolved and the relationships may not be totally severed, but can be integrated into the body of our experience so that it becomes less painful and part of our professional knowledge. This fits with the work of Klass, Silverman and Nickman (1996) and Walter (1999), which suggests that it is possible to hold our experiences while seeing them from different viewpoints and developing their coherence within our professional knowledge. This requires considerable skill and detachment.

Talking it through

The immediate shock of loss is followed by the need to work through the experience, make sense of it, build it into our career story and learn from it. This involves telling, retelling and gradually crafting our story of the experience. For most people this is best done with feedback from those they respect and trust and this can be a reciprocal learning experience. Those who were part of the experience, especially the bereaved mother, also play a key part.

Lamers (1997) and Parkes (2002) consider the importance of healthcare professionals conversing openly with one another regarding their feelings about death. They conclude that without such honest and frank discourse no individual could ever be truly sensitive to the needs of others. Cutler (1998) and Spencer (1994) identify that nurses may often be conscious of words and actions at the time of a death, but they rarely took time out to reflect on how they felt, or indeed to try to make sense of why they had particular feelings at different times. Our work supports Cutler (1998) and Spencer (1994), in that some of the midwives also had difficulty vocalising their feelings. Other midwives were able to articulate their feelings of professional grief.

The crafting of painful stories requires a safe setting. Some midwives talked over their experiences with family members and close friends. We know this is a means of coping widely used in midwifery (Kirkham, Morgan and Davies 2006), though it raises concerns for both confidentiality and the midwife's professional coping when she loses key personal supporters. Other midwives avoided discussing their work with family or friends to protect their immediate circle; two felt they could not discuss stillbirths with their partner because of their own infertility problems. This left them very isolated if they also lacked professional confidants.

A strong ethos of sharing though conversation, as a means of negotiating the meaning of professional grief, helped some of the midwives studied. Junior midwives valued listening to the experience of more senior midwives in the hope that they could learn ways to handle and learn from their own experiences. Those midwives who saw the sharing of experiences as therapeutic were active in promoting group or individual discussions. Such discussions were reported as helping colleagues to put into words the meaning they attached to events around a stillbirth and their part in that tragedy. However, not all midwives were skilled in putting their feelings into words; many lacked the opportunity to do so or were too anxious to create such opportunities. None of the NHS midwives saw such opportunities as built into the practice of their workplace.

Our studies show it is important for midwives to choose who they talk to about loss. The listener must be right for them in terms of their clinical and personal experience and their perceived empathy and trustworthiness. They also need considerable skill to perform this role most usefully. Those who worked with a clinical partner or in a small team, as community midwives or IMs, spoke of trusting their colleagues and discussing their experiences with them, though this may not always be the case (Deery 2003; Deery and Kirkham 2007). Those who had flexibility in their working lives, again mainly community midwives and IMs, made considerable efforts to seek out the right person with whom to talk. But most midwives work in hospitals, most stillbirths take place in hospitals and hospital midwives had the most difficulty in this respect, both in finding the right colleague to talk with and in accessing the bereaved mother to talk with her.

Some of the midwives interviewed needed more skilled support. One had paid for psychotherapy and others for counselling for themselves; others could probably have benefited from professional help.

Supervision

Several of the midwives interviewed felt that the supervision of midwives is developing in ways that could provide support around grief and loss. Few had experienced such support from supervisors though one worked hard to provide it as a supervisor.

Some of the respondents did not see a supervisor as an acceptable person with whom to discuss their experiences around stillbirth. The strength of this belief correlated with the midwives' feelings of culpability and guilt. They were very aware of the supervisor's role in policing midwifery practice and therefore could not acknowledge any vulnerability to her.

Where the supervisor suspended the midwife during investigation of the death, the midwives equated the suspension with a pronouncement of their guilt, which was internalised in the isolation that ensued.

Guilt and self-blame

Self-blame seems common amongst women, even in situations where they are abused (e.g. Garratt 2010), and is certainly common amongst midwives (Kirkham 1999; Deery and Kirkham 2007). Midwives in our study spoke of their guilt and self-blame. Where they could discuss their feelings with others who would challenge this view, it was possible for guilt and self-blame to be resolved. This was not possible in some cases and continuing self-blame left some midwives in a vulnerable emotional state and prevented them from handling their experience so as to benefit themselves and their future clients.

Johns (2004), reflecting on his work in palliative care, states that 'being guilty is a form of self-abuse'. In his view 'our caring selves are too valuable to beat up' and he stresses our primary responsibility to care for ourselves (145). Nevertheless, our socialisation as women, reinforced by training and practise as NHS midwives, makes guilt a hard habit to break. Many mothers feel guilt after a stillbirth (Klaus and Kennell 1982). Self-blame is common in bereaved mothers who feel that their body let their baby down (e.g. Fahey-McCarthy 2003) and this can be seen in many societies (Cecil 1996). Writing of her own stillbirth, McCracken (2009) sees such blame as 'a compulsive behaviour' (142), which can 'accomplish nothing' (142). This analogy is very powerful for bereaved mothers and midwives, since compulsive behaviours are notoriously difficult to change.

Responsibility and guilt are very different and it seems important to move beyond the compulsive state of guilt to take responsibility for healing the pain of loss and for using our sad experiences to develop our practice. In order to do this, we have to examine, rather than simply justify, our responses. This requires a degree of openness and vulnerability, which can feel very unsafe in the modern NHS. Midwives often found they lacked the resources to do this.

STORIES

Storytelling is important in midwifery (Olafsdottir and Kirkham 2009; Jordan 1993; Barclay *et al.* 2005) and an appropriate repertoire of stories can inform a secure basis for both clinical decision-making and the education of pregnant women and student midwives.

After a traumatic experience there is a need to rebuild our professional story; to create a coherence with which we can work, to restore 'the continuity of meaning' (Marris 1996: 48) contained within our professional life. Stories are our individual ways of viewing life events. Viewpoints can change as stories develop and other viewpoints can be admitted. Riches and Dawson (2000) recommend that 'one must recognise the power of stories and suspend judgement on people's reactions to their grief' (186). Sense making continues over developing iterations, for the teller and for hearers (Allan, Fairtlough and Heinzen 2002). For the midwives we interviewed their continuity of professional meaning was expressed in their need to show themselves as caring and competent and/or learning practitioners even in tragic situations.

Our data show that pride in giving good care after a death was important in the midwife's story and as a consolation the midwife could offer the mother when she felt she had nothing else to give. Where the midwife responsible for the birth also gave postnatal care, this offered the potential for a positive role in the mother and family's journey through grief. Thus, efforts to deal with their grief could be reciprocal. Where care was fragmented these possibilities were not present.

The midwives expressed a need for their own efforts and care to become a positive part of the mother's story. They had to hear this from the mother. It was therefore important to see her again and to hear from her that the care given around the still-birth was appreciated. Where it was possible, midwives valued having an ongoing part in the story of the mother and family postnatally, and expressing their grief in words and actions, such as by attending funerals, helped them to deal with their grief. Cards and letters from bereaved parents were particularly valued as evidence of the midwife's positive part in the mother's story. The reciprocal relationship between the mother's story of her loss and that of the midwife was very important to the IMs as they were involved with the families for considerable periods of time after the stillbirth. On occasions these entwined stories developed over years and future pregnancies and demonstrated how stories can continue to develop positively and professional learning can develop further over time. This was in sharp contrast to the stories of some of the hospital midwives who could not see the mother again after the birth. These stories appeared frozen in time and embodied shock, guilt and blame, which continued to be painful for the midwives and could damage working relationships with colleagues.

To build their stories so as to resolve grief and learn professionally, midwives expressed two needs. Firstly, they needed sufficient control over their own practice to give what they saw as good care. Where they were instructed to undertake other tasks which prevented this, they felt powerless and guilty and grieved for the good practice they could not give. They were also fearful that the mother saw them as neglectful when she was most vulnerable. Secondly, they needed appropriate support so they could talk and reflect on their experiences safely. Some found this support in their own social circle, some talked with supportive colleagues and a few found skilled professional help. Others held the memory unresolved, lacking confidants amongst their colleagues and avoiding such discussion outside work so as to protect family and friends. For them the memory stayed as a painful emotional scar, though some gained from this a determination to prevent this happening to colleagues.

RECIPROCITY

Studies of caseload midwifery have demonstrated the reciprocal relationships that develop over time with continuity of carer and the mutually sustaining potential of these relationships between mothers and midwives and amongst midwifery colleagues (McCourt and Stevens 2009; Stevens 2003). The key factor here is the development of trust over time as the midwife's loyalty moves from her employer towards her client (Brodie 1996) and the developing relationship erodes the power difference between professional and client (Marris 1996). In these circumstances, the midwife and mother can invest their energy and skills in a relationship that they know will continue. Relationships with a small group of colleagues with similar work practices and values can develop in parallel with relationships with clients.

Our studies extend the research findings concerning reciprocity and continuity of midwifery care into dealing with grief. The giving of good care, respectful and sensitive to individual needs, together with supportive listening to each other's developing stories, was experienced as enabling for mothers and midwives where the circumstances of care allowed mutual trust to develop over time. The sustained caring, which some hospital midwives linked with vulnerability, could, in these circumstances 'nourish and sustain' midwives, who thereby achieved 'a fine balance' (Johns 2004: 149).

The reciprocal relationship between the mother's developing story of her loss and that of the midwife was striking in the narratives of the IMs, as was their ability, together, to transform their painful loss into an experience that, while always tragic, could also be enabling.

Reciprocal relationships with colleagues also helped midwives in the immediate circumstances of grief and later in seeking to make sense of their experience. Some hospital midwives were fortunate in having empathic colleagues, but most of the narratives of mutual support amongst colleagues came from community and independent midwifery. This may be because of smaller working teams or partnerships, or it may be because more flexible working conditions enabled the midwives to seek support for themselves more effectively as well as to give ongoing support to their clients. Mutual support networks certainly seemed to be much better developed by midwives who worked outside hospitals.

Thus, in contexts that supported nurturing, midwives experienced reciprocity between positive relationships with clients and with colleagues. These relationships could support and develop each other, creating a positive spiral. In contexts that were more task orientated and where care was fragmented, a vicious circle of blame and guilt was reported.

BALANCING ENGAGEMENT AND DETACHMENT

Some of the hospital midwives interviewed preferred giving care to bereaved women with whom they did not already have a relationship. They expressed some reserve about getting too close to the women's pain and wished to give good care with minimal pain to themselves. One hospital midwife stated that knowing the mother before the labour increased the guilt she felt after the stillbirth. This is the same group of midwives with the greatest problems with regard to support in grief. The midwives who knew their clients and provided continuity of care found that within those relationships they could work through their grief alongside the mother, and they had the consolations of providing good ongoing care and colleague support.

Midwives' skill in balancing engagement with detachment is important for them and for their clients (Deery and Hunter 2010). There is substantial evidence that meaningful relationships are crucial for midwives and mothers (Hunter *et al.* 2008; Deery and Hunter 2010).

We know that women want midwives who will relate to them, not 'uncaring encounters' with midwives who are 'absently present' (Berg *et al.* 1996). Mothers value midwives who listen as well as checking their clinical condition (Edwards 2005). To relate well, midwives need to constantly 'move and mediate in a sensitive and flexible manner between closeness and detachment' (Deery and Hunter 2010: 49).

This ensures that our clients can feel supported while exercising autonomy and without becoming overdependent. Maintaining this balance, which Johns (2004) likens to a dance, is a dynamic process that requires skill and reciprocity between the midwife and the mother.

This balance ensures that midwives are sensitive to their own emotional needs (Carmack 1997) and maintain sufficient detachment to observe the impact of their care upon their different clients. Yet so many of the ways of coping seen in hospitals, such as the denial of emotion by their medical colleagues that midwives reported, or stereotyping women (Kirkham *et al.* 2002) or fragmented care (Menzies Lyth 1988) or dissociation (Garratt 2010), serve to unbalance us in the long term, taking the pleasure out of the job and serving to deprive women of our focused attention and listening. Relationship gives satisfaction and confidence to mothers and midwives; yet most of our coping reactions, while saving time and defending us from anxiety, also 'defend' us from relationship and thereby impoverish all concerned.

Two community midwives spoke of their need for professional boundaries when giving care to bereaved mothers for prolonged periods. Their colleagues helped with their other work, but not with the grief they felt as a result of providing care for these women (*see* Chapter 5). The way in which these midwives spoke of their need for boundaries was similar to the way some midwives spoke of their containment of grief, so as not to impose it upon those near to them. Both responses were logical in a context of professional isolation and vulnerability, but they are damage limitation strategies rather than moves towards healing and professional growth. Boundaries may be needed, but there is a real danger that they become permanent barriers 'that keep others out or keep the self in' (Johns 2004: 151) rather than part of the dynamic balance of constantly developing skills. The IMs, who had built good support networks for themselves, did not speak of boundaries, though they gave the impression that their boundaries, like their comfort zones, were wider than those of their NHS colleagues. They certainly provided postnatal support for much longer and made themselves more easily available to their clients.

It is crucial that midwives know the limits of their skills in supporting bereaved women and when and to whom to refer such women for further help. This subject did not come up in the data, because we were addressing midwives' responses not those of mothers. It is equally important that we know the limits of our skills in self-care. A few IMs sought professional help in dealing with the impact of these cases upon them. A degree of detachment and self-awareness is needed in deciding when the midwife has reached the limit of her skills and where specialised professional help is needed by the midwife or the mother.

Midwives can best learn the dynamic balance of engagement and detachment within relationships with colleagues who are accepted as good professional role models clinically or in supervision. In interaction with such colleagues they are likely also to observe the degree of detachment needed to suspend judgement and thereby reflect upon and learn from experiences.

Balance between engagement and detachment is learned from good role models and practised with a degree of autonomy and control of working time. In pressured and increasingly standardised hospital practice, none of these factors may be available to midwives and they may also witness a rush to judge caregivers.

SUGGESTIONS FOR THE CREATION OF A FRAMEWORK OF SUPPORT FOR MIDWIVES WHO ARE INVOLVED WITH STILLBIRTH

Stillbirth documentation

We know that the initial numbness and bewilderment of grief can impact upon memory. The impact of stillbirth upon a midwife is likely to increase the likelihood of clerical error or omission in the vast amount of documentation required. In this study, two midwives considered that the trauma of a sudden stillbirth impaired their clerical accuracy. They were both formally censored by their supervisor of midwives.

Several of the midwives reported their fear of inaccuracy or omissions in stillbirth documentation and the resulting summons to a clinical manager's or their midwifery supervisor's office. Later, midwives reported their mounting anxiety as to whether their record keeping was of sufficient quality to protect them in the perinatal mortality meeting concerning the case. They experienced these meetings as occasions for blame rather than learning, and approached them in fear and dread. The fear associated with stillbirth documentation can thus be considerably prolonged. Fear as well as grief can have a negative effect upon the memory and clerical accuracy, creating a vicious circle of anxiety and potential error in documentation.

The perceived additional stress of completing the stillbirth documentation as well as supporting the mother may, as our data have highlighted, result in some midwives finding ways of reducing the number of intrauterine deaths and subsequent stillbirth cases for which they are willing to care. Such decisions may spring from a need for self-care rather than professional intimidation or lack of sensitivity. The practice of such self-care, which is observed as seeking to pass the buck, may be quite wide spread (Cutler 1998; Crookes 1996).

The additional psychological trauma that followed errors in documentation may have been prevented if local practice and/or policy required the scrutiny of all stillbirth documentation by a colleague for comprehensiveness and accuracy, before the attending midwife handed over care. If such a practice of supervising documentation completion existed, each midwife would feel helped and supported, irrespective of personal emotions present at the time of the stillbirth. It would then not be incumbent on the midwife to request assistance; it would be a simple expression of a collective understanding of the impact of loss.

Practical help

Offering to give some care to the bereaved mother can help the midwife immensely, both by giving her the chance of a restorative break and acknowledging the painful nature of working with the bereaved. Sometimes that acknowledgement alone can prevent the midwife from feeling isolated and burdened with the emotional weight of her work. Such sharing can be helpful to the helper too, in developing her support skills within short and manageable interactions. Midwives were also grateful when colleagues took on their other work so that they could concentrate on the bereaved mother. Much more of this latter help was reported rather than the former.

The taking of tissues samples from a stillborn baby is without doubt an unenviable task. One midwife noted the positive impact of being supported by a colleague during the undertaking of that procedure. Another expressed great distress and anxiety at having no support from her colleagues while completing this requirement. The help of a pathologist or laboratory technician to teach the skill of tissue sampling may be useful, but at the time the support of a colleague is needed. Support for the midwife concerned should be forthcoming from other midwives without request, in recognition of the emotional and sensitive personal feelings such a task may engender.

Similarly, a midwife, irrespective of seniority, may find the handling of a macerated stillborn baby a difficult experience. It is an experience that few healthcare professionals other than a midwife will face. There is little one can do to prepare any midwife for the uncomfortable nature of that task. However, if an environment of emotional safety can be generated where midwives can acknowledge their feelings, irrespective of status, this may result in more midwives feeling confident to request support from colleagues at a time when they feel vulnerable.

Caring for a woman in labour with a known intrauterine death involves considerable emotion work for the midwife. Providing care at the same time for a woman expecting a live birth involves a degree of emotional gymnastics, which we do not think should be expected of any midwife. Such allocation of work, inevitably, neglects the needs of all those concerned and can be profoundly damaging to them.

The opportunity to reflect and the skills required

There are many circumstances in which it is a valid choice to put our own feelings on one side, especially when attending to the needs of clients. Hiding our feelings from ourselves is rarely wise. Such repression of grief experiences 'traps our precious energy and gives our buried emotions even more power over us' (Friedeberger 1996: xii). Acknowledging our grief, anger and fear is a start towards understanding and acceptance and requires skills that can be developed.

There are various processes by which difficult emotional experiences can be used as learning opportunities. Within NHS midwifery such processes may be unknown or resisted (Deery 2003; Deery and Kirkham 2007) because of the anxieties engendered. It is therefore clear that processes can only be recommended where the midwife feels safe to explore the painful feelings involved.

The ultimate safety from external threat may be experienced in private writing. Bolton has shown how this can be done to very good effect as 'Reflective Practice' (2001) or as creative writing (1999). Journal writing can be painful because of the degree of honesty it requires; but it can also be self-affirming (Johns 2004). Machin (2009: 68–70) details the gains that can flow from keeping a journal and reading the writings of others experiencing grief in similar circumstances. Sarton, as a poet and novelist, wrote of skills that can benefit us all, though we will not all produce great literature.

> [W]e may learn a devise for discharging tension and apprehensions which we might otherwise not have strength to bear, and which as it is, become simply transposable *energy*. So grief itself is transposed into a curious joy.
>
> (1980: 21, emphasis in the original)

Journal writing is a good way of detaching ourselves slightly from our emotions so we can examine them, without being bowled over by them, and then decide what we can learn from our experience. Meditation can serve the same purpose. '[E]ach opens the possibility of looking at whatever comes up, and reflecting on it without getting involved in it. Both practices develop detachment, and bring clarity, acceptance and peace' (Friedeberger 1996: 173).

A degree of detachment is essential if we are to step back from our experience sufficiently to examine it and see if we could do better. This is utterly different from the dissociation (Garratt 2010), which keeps us emotionally separate from experience that is too painful to handle and which serves to hide that experience and to cut us off from others with whom we might share it.

Skills of detachment and reflection can be practised and developed in solitude, or verbally in a group with ground rules to help members feel safe. There is a considerable amount of literature on the techniques of reflective practice in nursing (e.g. Johns 2000, 2002, 2004). Group reflection brings the potential for personal support and cross-fertilisation of ideas. A similar basis underlies clinical supervision, which can be a one to one experience or undertaken in a group. Clinical supervision is uncommon in midwifery and may be experienced as threatening and therefore be resisted (Deery 2003). There are some examples of successful clinical supervision in midwifery. Clinical supervision has been practised in groups for some years in the neonatal unit in Exeter (Derbyshire 2000). It is noteworthy that neonatal care is an area where death is relatively common. Their practice of clinical supervision is grounded in the belief that

> [q]uality in patient care is not achieved by decree, nor by striving to reach standards set by others. Rather, it is achieved by the endless pursuit, by each individual practitioner, of greater understanding and better practice.
>
> (Derbyshire 2000: 172)

Jones set up a process of guided reflection for midwives, facilitated by a supervisor of midwives, as a fundamental practice in a new birth centre. At first some midwives tended to continue with practices rooted in the hospital consultant unit with which they felt comfortable but which did not necessarily reflect the philosophy of the birth centre. Following discussion of one birth, it was encouraging when a midwife commented, 'I didn't know that before; I think I would manage the situation differently next time' (Jones 2000: 161).

This process was experienced as empowering, providing opportunities for debriefing and learning together 'as the story of a birth unfolds' (Jones 2000: 162).

It took time for midwives to become confident in group reflection, to accept critical enquiry as non-judgemental and to trust each other in terms of confidentiality and support.

> *It would be unrealistic to say that nobody's feelings are ever hurt because sometimes this causes inevitable pain. We all care deeply that what we do is right so realising that there could be a better way causes us discomfort . . . these are growing pains and far preferable to the anaesthetised routine that has always been good enough.*
>
> (midwife, quoted in Jones 2000: 162)

It is noteworthy that this took place in a birth centre, with a small constant group of colleagues with whom trust could be developed.

To learn the skills of reflection, midwives have to feel safe enough to let go of the anxieties that hold them back (another parallel with the experience of their clients [Anderson 2010]) and open themselves to the possibilities of change with all its 'growing pains'. This is unlikely to be achieved anew in the presence of professional grief. Where the habits of reflection and a trusted group of reflective practitioners already exist they provide a supportive context for the resolution of grief and learning from sad experience. The habits of attention, patience, suspension of judgement, active listening and reflection are like muscles, in that they can be developed with practise. Then 'what begins as a necessary exercise gradually becomes natural. And then immense landscapes open out in front of you' (Garner 1996: 12).

Student midwives need to learn the habits of reflection and of giving and receiving support. This practice may be at odds with those they see in their clinical placements and therefore needs to be modelled in some part of their practice as well as formally taught. Fahy-McCarthy, a midwife teacher and mother of a stillborn baby, describes reflection to students as 'entering a counselling relationship with "self"' (2003: 602). Such an ongoing relationship is self-nurturing as well as enabling grief to be integrated into one's professional practice. As well as learning the habits of reflection, which will sustain them in many different situations, student midwives need the opportunity to consider death and grief and their place in midwifery practice (Kenworthy 2004). Since many are motivated to become midwives because they see it as a happy area of work, it is important that its tragic aspects are considered before they are met in clinical practice (Mander 2006).

Reflection, in private or with others, requires 'transference from feeling to thinking, a conscious exploration' of our experience through 'unremitting ruthless analysis' (Sarton 1980: 43). Most of the NHS midwives interviewed, together with many in other studies (e.g. Deery 2003), did not feel safe enough with each other to move from self-protection to self-analysis. Cultural change would be needed to achieve this in the context of NHS maternity hospitals.

While it is possible for the behaviour of individuals to change systems, change is easier to achieve with identified change agents. Support in coping with loss could be facilitated by supervisors of midwives or by designated bereavement midwives, if this was acknowledged to be a major part of their role and organised in such a way as not to overburden those individuals. However, such designation requires a commitment to cultural change.

CHAPTER 11

Loss in midwifery: the wider context and ways forward

BEING WITH WOMAN

The support skills needed around loss by both mothers and midwives are rooted in basic midwifery skills. As we worked on this book, we came to see how the need for these skills around loss highlights both the value we place upon being with women when they are very vulnerable and the difficulty in practising these skills in the context of modern maternity services.

Midwives have wide experience of being a quietly supportive presence, using their manner and well-chosen words to assure women that they can achieve what presently seems impossible. Such a presence is exactly what grieving midwives themselves need.

Helping women to live with uncertainty and 'embracing uncertainty together' with them is a key midwifery skill (Leap 2010). It is not a skill that maternity services in general are good at and, as the management of risk has been increasingly emphasised in recent years, the skills of living with what cannot be managed have been somewhat overlooked. Fortunately some midwives excel in these skills. After a baby dies both parents and carers 'may need to be supported in learning to live with contradiction and with that which cannot be explained' (Fahy-McCarthy 2003: 602).

Listening to women is a fundamental skill if midwifery is to focus on the individual woman. Actively listening to a woman is very difficult (Gilham 2000), especially in an institutional setting where there is great pressure to reduce the woman's personal story to a standardised clinical history. This leads women to see midwives as 'checking not listening' (Edwards 2005), which makes relationship, and all it can achieve, impossible. Checking is important but so is listening. Similarly, checking that all the tasks around stillbirths are completed is a start to supporting a midwife caring for a bereaved mother. Later, listening to her story validates her experience and supports her personal and professional development.

Attentive observation is vital in midwifery: in awareness of clinical observations that may give cause for concern or the observation of social or emotional cues that may suggest that a mother needs particular support. Similarly, attentive self-observation is needed by the midwife. Self-awareness enables her to monitor the impact of her care upon the mother. It also helps with professional trauma and grief, for when the feelings associated with an experience have been drawn out, examined, accepted and integrated into our body of knowledge, healing takes place. For mothers and for midwives, such observation must feel kind, gentle and not judgemental. Mothers and midwives deserve respect and gentle treatment.

Midwives are part of the birth, not just of babies and placentae, but also of mothers' birth stories. Whether deliberately seeking to debrief a mother, or in the normal course of postnatal care, midwives hear the early tentative tellings of the birth story. Careful observations, such as 'weren't you brave' or 'you did so well' or a remark to the father such as 'you must be so proud of her', can gently turn a developing story from one of passivity into one of empowerment. On the other hand, negative attitudes of midwives and obstetricians can have a negative effect upon women's self-image (Waldenstrom 2003; Simkin 1996), which increases in significance over time. The skills of being with woman develop with practise and can be developed further and more easily where continuity of care allows time for relationship and trust to develop. In modern fragmented, rushed and under-resourced hospital care it is harder to develop such skills, but they are still the heart of midwifery.

Midwives are very aware of how mothers differ in their responses to events around childbearing: what is clinically recorded as a normal delivery can be a traumatic experience and with appropriate care surgical intervention may be seen by the mother as enabling. Similarly, midwives differ in their responses to trauma. It is important therefore that no assumptions are made that the midwife can operate successful coping strategies at the time or after a death. Midwives also differ greatly as to when they wish to discuss their experiences and a listening ear needs to be available when they feel ready.

The emotion work of midwifery is best practised in a safe setting. We all know that trust is contagious and where a midwife trusts a mother, this can enable the mother to grow into trusting her body and herself. Mistrust is also contagious, whether between midwife and mother or amongst colleagues because of unspoken blame attributed in a previous tragedy. Fear is similarly contagious and hospitals are often experienced as fearful places. Mothers report this (Robinson 2003) and midwives in our studies were fearful of blame and judgement from colleagues, supervisors and management. Perinatal mortality meetings generated further tension in midwives, which mounted as the meeting approached. None of the respondents considered these meetings as positive learning experiences that generated support for them as individuals or even acknowledged that they may have been emotionally affected by the stillbirths.

We know that continuing support can have a positive impact on the outcomes of care (Hodnett et al. 2007). The emotional skills involved in such support are subtle, varied and need to be sustained. The midwife's attention can enable the woman to feel that she is heard and her experience is validated. The nature of the midwife's presence, especially during labour, can be experienced as enabling or diminishing, depending on whether the midwife is 'emotionally present' (Berg 2002: 54) or just 'checking' (Edwards 2005) . The midwife herself has a parallel need to feel that her voice is heard and her feelings validated, especially after a traumatic and emotionally draining experience. Without the positive experience of being supported and heard herself, it is difficult for her to give to women what she herself has not experienced.

Gentle nurturing or mothering by colleagues helped several midwives to diffuse the anger that they felt at the time of a stillbirth. Such care resembled the mothering of the mother by the midwife to enable her to mother her baby (Taylor 2010). Many of the midwives interviewed did not experience such care and did not feel able to seek it out. Mothers similarly reported that they don't like to ask when midwives are 'so busy' or when they are seen to be preoccupied with clinical tasks (Edwards 2005; Kirkham and Stapleton 2001). Some midwives felt that supervision could be a source of such nurturing.

Support networks are very important for effective functioning as a mother or a midwife and mutual support is the essence of such networks. It has been suggested that helping women antenatally to build the support networks that will sustain them postnatally is one of the most important areas of midwifery work (Leap 2010). Similarly, midwives need support networks for difficult aspects of their professional work. Those midwives who had built strong, mutually sustaining support networks benefited greatly from them in times of professional grief.

The pressures of work in hospital and the fragmented nature of hospital care seem to have prevented many of the midwives interviewed from seeing the parallels between their own needs and those of their clients or the potential for reciprocity in relationships with clients and colleagues. Nevertheless, they showed considerable insight into the needs of bereaved parents and were willing to experience blame and grief themselves to help meet those needs. The fragmented nature of their work produced fragmented coping strategies such as sealing off their own grief and finding nowhere to discuss it. Where midwives were involved with clients' needs over time, they seemed more aware of their own needs and planned to meet them.

Rothman (1996) states that

> [b]irth is not only about making babies. Birth is also about making mothers – strong, competent, capable mothers who trust themselves and know their inner strength.
>
> (253)

Given the striking parallels between the fundamental midwifery skills, which enable mothers, and the skills needed to support grieving midwives, a very similar statement could be made for midwives. Where skilled and appropriate support is available with relationships of trust, mothers and midwives can become increasingly strong, competent and capable.

THE CULTURE

NHS maternity services are both hierarchical and bureaucratic. Distinctions have been made between enabling and coercive bureaucracies (Adler and Borys 1996). However, the midwives we interviewed did not respond to the bureaucracies within which they worked as being enabling, and on stressful occasions they were fearful of doing the wrong thing, or omitting required tasks. Within hierarchical organisations, there is considerable pressure towards submission to authority. The pressures towards obedience and conformity in midwifery have been demonstrated and these pressures 'create conflict between the midwives' knowledge of how they would prefer to behave and concern to please authority and fit into the social group' (Hollins Martin and Bull 2008: 504). Such behaviour is called 'groupthink' by Allan, Fairtlough and Heinzen (2002), who see it as a situation where group cohesion is the main aim and fear of disagreement overrides commitment to the group's task. This makes it difficult for midwives to initiate change or to focus on the needs of their clients, despite the policy documents that advocate this. Moves towards the standardisation of services tend to exacerbate this situation.

This culture is also one of fear and blame. A Canadian GP obstetrician, Vania Jimenez, writes of 'the muzak of fear', constant in the background of modern obstetrics (quoted in Vadeboncoeur 2010: 35). Robinson (2003), from a maternity services consumer viewpoint, speaks of 'fear of loss of control, loss of power and loss of dominance. The inflexible system in which they have had to work for so long does not allow them to respond in any other way' (719). Allan, Fairtlough and Heinzen (2002) observe of the NHS in general that 'the culture appears to be one of blame and fear – and low learning. Individuals are expected to take responsibility but are not trusted or supported' (107). In such a context it is difficult to learn from our experiences beyond the obvious lessons of conformity and appearing competent.

Within this wider context, the culture of midwifery in the NHS is one of service and self-sacrifice (Kirkham 1999). While the motivation for such self-sacrifice can be high, such a culture can easily become one of self-neglect or even self-abuse (Johns 2004: 145). In an area of practice that requires skilled emotion work, self-neglect can limit our ability to respond to the needs of our clients and colleagues as well as ourselves. Over time it also creates a situation where midwives feel drained and dumped on; with no opportunity to recycle the 'emotional toxic waste' they have accumulated (Deery and Kirkham 2007) burnout is likely to follow. In these circumstances positive emotional energy can be seen as a finite resource, which is drained from midwives by the care they give without the possibility of the 'autonomous use of self that is pleasurable and satisfying in itself' (Deery and Hunter 2010).

Within the NHS, midwives feel very pressed for time. Stevens (2003) describes time as 'the ultimate control' for midwives. The tasks that must be completed have increased in number. In a business model of care, time is money, and tasks must be completed with speed and efficiency. People who are pressed for time cannot relate well. There are two responses to this: we can change the system of care, or we can reduce the tasks that need completing. Both options are promising.

The rigidity of NHS maternity services cannot be appropriate in a modern society that values choice and flexibility. Those of us within maternity services have had to be flexible in accommodating unprecedented change in recent years. Yet despite official rhetoric, the flexibility to nurture clients and staff when their need is greatest seems difficult to achieve, at least in this country. Despite the great pressures to conform and the muzak of fear, we need to accept that the culture within which we work in NHS maternity services is dysfunctional.

THE POSSIBILITY OF CULTURAL CHANGE

The extent to which midwives and their clients experience loss and grief means that it would be useful to make sense of grief at an organisational as well as a personal level. Finding the means to address this problem would offer the solution to many others.

The amount of change in recent years shows the extent to which change is possible. At a personal level, some of the midwives interviewed demonstrated this in endeavouring to prevent other midwives from suffering the isolation in grief that they had experienced. Role models are very powerful and can model positive change. The mutual support of IMs also shows what can be accomplished.

Supervision of midwives

Specific changes can help to move away from a culture of blame. The provision of good support for midwives who are suspended during a supervisory investigation following a death could do much to prevent isolation and self-blame. Formal apologies where their practice is vindicated would do much to prevent bitterness in these cases. For these and all midwives experiencing professional grief, the opportunity to talk without risk of blame would help those who speak and those who listen. Skilful drawing out of key issues in these stories could lead to greater support for midwives, which could prevent the more painful long-term consequences of grief. If such facilitation was included in the role of supervisors of midwives or specialist bereavement midwives, many midwives would be helped and skills with great clinical relevance would be modelled and experienced.

Stories as transformative

To achieve an acknowledgement of grief and stress as part of practice that should not be suppressed, a culture of openness is needed. If stories of grief and loss are to be told, a culture of storytelling is also needed. It is interesting that some management writers (e.g. Allan, Fairtlough and Heinzen 2002; Hampden-Turner 1990) see openness and the telling of professional stories as a way out of the inevitable dilemmas generated within organisations. 'Rule enforcement hides conflicts. Openness brings them out for everyone to see, to understand and to reframe' (Allan, Fairtlough and Heinzen 2002: 103–4). Malby and Pattison (1999), looking at the NHS, think that stories, over time, can produce positive organisational change.

To do this, a forum for storytelling is needed that must provide a safe, constructive and, ideally, a multi-professional setting. This is asking for a massive change in attitudes, but with commitment and role modelling from senior staff, this could be possible. If it seems impossible on a multi-professional level, we have precedents for the effectiveness of such practice within midwifery teams, with appropriate mentoring and small secure teams (e.g. Jones 2000; *see* Chapter 10). Such teams, with an appropriate degree of autonomy, do work in birth centres and have been created to provide continuity of care within large hospitals (Homer, Brodie and Leap 2001, 2008). Small groups of colleagues, working with appropriate ground rules, can provide the psychological safety, which is needed if learning is to take place in work teams (Edmondson 1999). They can become 'creative compartments' (Fairtlough 1994) within maternity services, which demonstrate how a consistent practice of openness creates trust and thus changes the culture of an organisation. Such teams would meet midwives' needs for both autonomy and support, as is already experienced in birth centres (Kirkham 2003), by IMs and in other 'Birth models that work' (Davis-Floyd *et al.* 2009). When a culture of reflection and openness is nurtured within midwifery, relationships with colleagues from other professions tend to improve, probably as a result of the greater confidence and improved communication skills of the midwives concerned (Kirkham 2003).

Where stories show conflicting values for instance – where medical colleagues objected to midwives showing emotion in the presence of their clients – the telling of both stories with examination of their underlying values and fears could lead to the creation of a story that subsumes both value sets (Allan, Fairtlough and Heinzen 2002). With goodwill and time, this should be possible. It would facilitate growth for all concerned and remove blame and ill-will springing from past unexamined differences. The reframing of the situation so that the two values of the dilemma are subsumed into a single, more fundamental, value would require very similar skills to those of reflection on our individual stories. Each practice would help the other.

Such practices would avoid the perils of groupthink, since the group's aims and purposes would have to be openly and rigorously examined to make sure that they are clear to everyone and there are no hidden reservations. Thus, our efforts to make sense of our stories would benefit the whole team, rather than just individuals, and skills and working relationships would be developed in the process.

The final stage of such dilemma resolution – the generation of support for the reframed value and building it into practice stories – is aimed to create a 'virtuous circle of support' for individuals as well as values (Allan, Fairtlough and Heinzen 2002). This would be infinitely better than the vicious circle of ineffective coping strategies reported so often by the midwives we interviewed. Such sessions to explore, examine and build stories might be more welcomed and more productive than perinatal mortality meetings.

Techniques to achieve openness

To achieve cultural change we need a degree of openness beyond the 'defensive routines' (Argyris 1990) that currently protect us and the flaws of our present system.

Some midwives achieve this through 'Nonviolent Communication' (Rosenberg 2003), which is a technique for focusing attention compassionately. It is structured around the observations, feelings, needs and requests of both parties in an inter-action. This structuring of response enables practitioners to cut through defensive responses and the habits that limit our attention to ourselves and others. Nonviolent Communication has had positive results in many organisational settings.

Some practitioners draw techniques for achieving open communication from various religious traditions. Johns (2004) uses Buddhist techniques of mindful-ness to reflect upon his work in palliative care, often adapting these to the Christian beliefs of his clients.

Another way of approaching this is through 'dialogue', an approach aimed at uncovering the common meaning in a group or an individual. 'The first task in cre-ating such shared meanings is simply to apprehend the meanings of others' (Dixon 1998: 30). There are a number of techniques for achieving this, according to Dixon, but the starting point for dialogue is always listening, as it should be for midwifery.

Really focusing on listening is rare; more often we are also thinking how we will respond, or what the speaker's words remind us of, or what we want to do next. Such active listening is tremendously affirming for the person heard, it can also achieve 'the softening up, the opening up, of the mind, and looking at all the opinions' (Bohm 1993). Such an approach enables us to overcome the limited, fragmented view we derive from working in fragmented systems. It is not about defending our own position and as such requires a degree of vulnerability in examining our own thoughts and feeling as well as those of others.

Such practice requires a safe setting, some degree of skill and 'hope that things can change' (Dixon 1998: 53) since hopelessness creates silence, or depression, not dialogue. It means that 'undiscussable' issues can be raised (Dixon 1998: 107). Dialogue can change relationships, even within hierarchies at work. It could pro-vide a focused and affirming context for telling and developing our stories. It could prevent the frozen resentment and distrust of colleagues, which some midwives described as following their experience of a stillbirth years before.

'Openness, like defensiveness, tends to be self-confirming' (Marris 1996: 115). Once midwives have the circumstances where they can experience a sense of control and understanding in their relationships and the skills to practise in dialogue with clients and colleagues, they are likely to go on developing those skills and circum-stances. This virtuous spiral has the potential to enhance the care of all concerned.

There are a range of practices and techniques we could use to change the culture of midwifery for the better. The skills required are very similar to the fundamental midwifery skills, though these may be in danger of being lost under the mounting technical and clerical tasks now required of midwives and the wider NHS pressures to compliance and conformity. We know that midwives wish to practice to the best of their ability and require a degree of autonomy in order to do this (Ball, Curtis and Kirkham 2002); they also need skills in active listening (Gilham 2000). Midwives suffering professional grief need the same skills. So, in a real sense, the support avail-able to mothers and midwives in grief acts as a touchstone for the whole maternity service. Without trust and safe space in which to talk, mothers cannot feel secure and a sensitive midwifery workforce is not sustainable. It is vital that we make good provision for midwives suffering loss, because they experience loss in many aspects of their professional experience.

OTHER LOSSES

We are aware of many other losses suffered by midwives, which produce professional grief akin to that following stillbirth and which could be helped by similar changes.

Maternal death

Mander's (2001, 2006) research on the impact of maternal death on midwives showed similar, but much more traumatic experiences, than those associated with stillbirth. The midwives involved formed an isolated 'in group' who felt they could not share their tragic experiences with others and who were often avoided by colleagues. Support made a crucial difference in this terrible situation, but was not always available; sometimes the avoidance extended to senior colleagues. Midwives were particularly dependent on colleague support in these circumstances as there was little possibility of their grief being validated by the family's story of the death or even of them knowing that story.

The extent of the shock midwives experienced when involved with maternal death showed the extent to which the midwives felt unprepared for both the death and for dealing with their own subsequent emotions.

Loss of accustomed work setting and relationships

A variety of clinical work settings are generally seen as essential experience for newly qualified midwives. As midwives become more experienced, most find their niche in a particular area of work (Kirkham, Morgan and Davies 2006). Fortunately midwives vary greatly in the niches that suit them best. A reasonable amount of variation in place of work is accepted as necessary to maintain skills. Where a shortage of midwives means that midwives are moved frequently and without notice to 'plug the gaps' in the service, they dislike this intensely. They report disruption of relationships with colleagues and clients (Ball, Curtis and Kirkham 2002). Midwives report frequent changes of workplace within one shift as highly disruptive. With pressure on resources, such disruption becomes increasingly common, resulting in high levels of loss of control and an inability to plan care for even a few hours ahead.

Centralisation of maternity services has lead to the closure of many 'small' maternity units, and hospitals are now being closed that would have been seen as large 10 years ago. Many midwives therefore suffer loss of the hospital at which they chose to work, as well as their immediate work setting within that service. For some this is linked with loss of a local service and many midwives have campaigned with local people to keep their maternity services. Where these closures go ahead, as they usually do, midwives experience considerable loss and grieve for the service they had. The extent of this loss is rarely acknowledged in orientating midwives to new centralised units and can be a factor in midwives leaving midwifery.

Their grief for the service lost can limit the extent to which midwives can embrace innovations in midwifery care. In a recent study of a birth centre that was set up following the amalgamation of two units into a large new hospital, those interviewed described the local midwives as 'mourning' the service they had lost and feeling 'bereft' and 'betrayed' (Deery, Hughes and Kirkham 2010). In such circumstances, the midwives could not accept the birth centre, seeing it as less than what they had lost and they did not want to work there. The innovation lacked support and, despite its good clinical outcomes and client satisfaction, it failed to thrive and ultimately closed. Many birth centres and midwife-led innovations in service have followed centralisations of services. Without the opportunity for staff to come to terms with their loss and grief, such innovations may well be neglected and unsupported.

Many changes in maternity services involve loss of colleague support for midwives. This may be because hospitals are closed, services reorganised or employees being frequently moved about. Relationships with colleagues have the potential to sustain midwives in their work and provide an important source of job satisfaction (Kirkham, Morgan and Davies 2006; Kirkham and Morgan 2006). These relationships take time and effort to develop and when trusted colleagues are no longer immediately available midwives suffer real loss. Midwives feel safest and work best with a small group of trusted colleagues. Where their work is organised so that they have an ever-changing army of colleagues, collegial relationships cannot be developed and midwives therefore experience lack of support.

Loss of autonomy

We know that the major reason midwives leave midwifery is because they cannot practice as they would wish (Ball, Curtis and Kirkham 2002). The present study echoes this in so far as the NHS midwives spoke of not being able to give the care they wished to give to bereaved mothers. A midwife who feels she cannot be the midwife she wants to be suffers loss of control within her work and loss of her professional sense of self.

There are many pressures towards conformity that limit midwives' autonomy. The current tendency to standardise care places a further limitation on midwives' freedom to respond to the needs of individual mothers, despite the policy rhetoric of maternal choice and woman-centred services (Department of Health 1993, 2004, 2007). The prevalence of bullying (RCM 1996; Gillen 2007) and horizontal violence (Leap 1997) as well as the pressures towards obedience (Hollins, Martin and Bull 2008), also limit midwives' autonomy.

Yet a degree of control within one's work is essential to occupational health.

> People who have jobs characterised by high demands and little control are more vulnerable to infectious disease, coronary heart disease, psychiatric disorders, hypertension, exhaustion, and alcohol and drug abuse. They are also just plain unhappier at work.
>
> (Taylor 2002: 173)

The contrast between the IMs and the NHS midwives we studied was striking in this regard. The IMs were potentially very isolated, yet they were able to organise their work so that they could pride themselves on the quality of the care they gave and develop optimum relationships with clients and colleagues. They clearly found their work fulfilling, though sad at times, and they had a highly developed mutual support network. The narratives of NHS midwives showed the same aims, but many expressed frustration with the limitations placed upon them. Their limited control over the care they gave also limited their learning and coping strategies, thus creating a vicious circle in terms of their capacity to cope with the emotion work, which is central to midwifery practice and self-care.

Personal loss

Loss in midwives' personal lives can also impact on their work. We are both aware of this from our own experiences of bereavement.

On the day my mother died, I (MK) was required to give an antenatal class in the evening. This seemed an impossible task but no colleague was available to help and I did not want to just put a notice on the door cancelling the class. I sat down with a heavy heart and told the expectant couples that the meaning of motherhood had changed totally for me on that day. The discussion that followed was of a level I have rarely encountered, covering fear of death and fetal abnormality as well as two mothers describing bereavements during their present pregnancy, which they felt they could not mention in previous sessions. Members of that group were amazingly supportive of me and of each other. They continued to meet for several years as a mutual support group and strong friendships were forged amongst them. I learned a lot in that session about the reciprocal effects of emotional openness as well as about topics that can usefully be covered in classes that I had not broached before. Autonomy and support helped me here. The setting felt safe both in the group and in my workplace: I had already met the group several times and my manager had repeatedly proved herself to be trustworthy.

Many midwives suffer loss with respect to their own health. We are both aware of the poignancy of colleagues' experiences when returning to work after a mastectomy and helping a new mother to breastfeed, or returning after a hysterectomy to assist at a birth. Such midwives need loving support from their colleagues if they are to use their own experience to improve their professional practice rather than walling off this painful area of their lives.

Bewley (2010) has researched midwives' childlessness and its impact upon their practice. When women in labour asked these midwives if they had children, this question could be very painful for them. Some even invented children to help them in this difficult situation and give them credibility in their clients' eyes. Mander (1996) reported her observations about the probing and personal nature of questions asked of child-free midwives, which echo the findings of previous writers (Bartlett 1994). She also recognised the well-documented negative stereotypes surrounding child-free women suggesting they are selfish, and somehow 'abnormal' (Bartlett 1994; Morrel 1994).

Some of Bewley's respondents reported depression after their loss but were reticent about disclosing this or any need for counselling or treatment because of the much publicised links between depression and the murders committed by nurses such as Beverly Allit (2010). These midwives adopted a professional façade, as they concealed aspects of their own experiences that might alarm their clients, or which might expose their own, sometimes very new and raw, feelings. Many participants expressed dismay that, despite the emphasis now placed on supporting bereaved parents, midwifery colleagues were often less than supportive to their peers. Many confirmed how they wanted to use what were potentially negative experiences to improve the outcome for others. They formed support groups, raised funds, updated literature in their own workplace to support parents and acquired specific knowledge that informed their work with their clients. Some shared their stories with clients, but there were mixed feelings, and some were unhappy with the outcome, and in some cases so were their clients. However, in order for midwives to be supportive, they need to be supported and nurtured themselves; this finding runs through so many studies of midwives' loss.

Clearly there are many ways in which good midwives can suffer loss that impacts upon their experience as midwives, just as Mander (2006) found many elements of loss in 'successful' childbearing. There are also striking similarities between their professional needs in the face of differing losses.

LEARNING FROM LOSS

Marris (1996) surveyed the literature and concluded that there are four conditions that influence whether an individual suffering loss will be able to work though grief successfully (*see* Chapter 2). Two of these conditions, childhood experience of attachment, and the opportunity to prepare for the loss, cannot be influenced by the midwife. Nevertheless, acknowledgement of the traumatic impact of sudden loss and nurturing of the individual concerned can help considerably. The other two of these conditions can be helped by midwives. Events after the loss can support the process of recovery, and midwives as individuals and at an organisational level can offer appropriate support. In the final condition, Marris (1996) states that 'the more conflicted, doubtful or unresolved' the meaning of what has been lost, the harder it is likely to be to reconstitute meaning (120).

For the midwives interviewed, restoring their continuity of professional meaning after loss could be fraught because of the dilemmas within their professional meaning before the loss. We know that midwives leave midwifery because they cannot practice as they would wish (Ball, Curtis and Kirkham 2002) but many midwives feel this and continue to practice (Kirkham, Morgan and Davies 2006). Some of the midwives we interviewed were deeply hurt by not being able to give the care they felt bereaved mothers needed and which they needed to give; others coped by adopting the defensive strategies of avoidance and isolation that they saw around them. Rigid hierarchical structures that depend upon but do not acknowledge relationships (Hunter *et al.* 2008), fragmented care, a climate of fear and a culture of self-sacrifice, together with a pressing need to appear to cope, prevented these midwives from acknowledging their needs or moving on from their experience. Like one of a couple who always fought but is bereft when widowed, the NHS midwives' relationship with their work before the loss showed elements of the problems that were vastly magnified by grief.

The difference between the responses to grief shown by independent and NHS midwives and between NHS midwives in hospital and community practice showed that the experience of grief could be greatly influenced by the immediate organisation of the workplace. The midwives interviewed showed considerable insight into the nature of grief and understanding of their clients' grief. The more controlled their work situation the less they were able to act upon their insights in terms of caring for their clients and themselves. The resulting feelings of helplessness prevented them from acting to resolve their grief that remained frozen as guilt, resentment or anger. Similarly, the tendency to avoid rather than help grieving colleagues left those colleagues isolated in their guilt and anger. These emotions have a corrosive effect on the individual over time and can inhibit further development of caring skills.

In many ways, midwives' experiences of loss highlight the problems within the organisation of midwifery care. Individual behaviour can make a big difference to colleagues' experiences of loss. Role models can be very powerful, but cultural change is also needed. Obedience to a system that is dysfunctional and could be so much better is not helping midwives to cope with loss, nor is it nurturing a sustainable workforce. Many aspects of modern midwifery reflect the uncertainties of the wider society (Bauman 2007) of which the NHS is part. Economic pressures also work against change (Baker 2005; Perkins 2004). Nevertheless, midwives and mothers can bring about change and are well placed to create precedents much needed throughout healthcare. We offer this book as an insight into the grief of midwives and the changes needed, so that the tragedies we are bound to experience do not produce the scars that can limit our future practice.

Bibliography

Adler PS, Borys B. (1996) Two types of bureaucracy: enabling and coercive. *Adm Sci Q.* **41**: 61–98.

Allan J, Fairtlough G, Heinzen B. (2002) *The Power of the Tale: using narratives for organisational success.* Chichester: John Wiley.

Anderson T. (2010) Feeling safe enough to let go: the relationship between a woman and her midwife during the second stage of labour. In: Kirkham M, editor. *The Midwife–Mother Relationship.* 2nd ed. Basingstoke: Macmillan. pp. 116–43.

Argyris C. (1990) *Overcoming Organisations Defences: facilitating organisational learning.* Boston, MA: Allyn and Bacon.

Baker M. (2005) Childbirth practices, medical intervention and women's autonomy: safer childbirth or bigger profits? *Women's Health and Urban Life.* **4**(2): 27–44.

Ball L, Curtis P, Kirkham M. (2002) *Why Do Midwives Leave?* London: Royal College of Midwives.

Barclay L, Aiavao F, Fenwick J, *et al.* (2005) *Midwives Tales: stories of traditional and professional birthing in Samoa.* Nashville, TN: Vanderbilt University Press.

Bartlett J. (1994) *Will You Be Mother? Women who choose to say no.* London: Virago.

Bauman Z. (2007) *Liquid Times: living in an age of uncertainty.* Cambridge, UK, and Malden, MA: Polity.

Benoliel JQ. (1988) Healthcare delivery: not conducive to teaching palliative care. *J Palliat Care.* **4**: 41–2.

Berg M. (2002) *Genuine Caring in Caring for the Genuine: childbearing and high risk as experienced by women and midwives.* Uppsala: Acta Universitatis Upsaliensis.

Berg M, Lundgren I, Hermansson E, *et al.* (1996) Women's experiences of the encounter with the midwife during childbirth. *Midwifery.* **12**: 11–15.

Bewley C. (2010) Midwives personal experiences and their relationships with women: midwives without children and midwives who have experienced pregnancy loss. In: Kirkham M, editor. *The Midwife–Mother Relationship.* 2nd ed. Basingstoke: Macmillan. pp. 190–207.

Bohm D. (1993) For trust try dialogue. *Resurgence.* **156**(13): 10–13.

Bolton G. (1999) *The Therapeutic Potential of Creative Writing: writing myself.* London: Jessica Kingsley.

——. (2001) *Reflective Practice: writing and professional development.* London: Paul Chapman.

Bowlby J. (1973) *Separation: anxiety and anger.* Vol. II of *Attachment and Loss.* New York, NY: Basic Books.

——. (1991) *Loss: sadness and depression.* Vol. III of *Attachment and Loss.* Harmondsworth: Penguin.

Boyle FM. (1997) *Mothers Bereaved by Stillbirth, Neonatal Death or Sudden Infant Death Syndrome.* Aldershot: Ashgate Press.

Brodie P. (1996) Australian team midwives in transition. *The Proceedings of the International Confederation of Midwives 24th Triennial Congress,* 26–31 May; Oslo: ICM, 132–4.

Bull P. (2001) State of the art: nonverbal communication. *The Psychologist.* 14(12): 644–7.

Burns N, Grove SK. (1995) *Understanding Nursing Research.* Philadelphia, PA: WB Saunders.

Canine JD. (1996) *The Psychosocial Aspects of Death and Dying.* Stanford, CT: Appleton and Lange.

Carmack BJ. (1997) Balancing engagement and detachment in caregving. *Image J Nurs Sch.* 29(2): 139–43.

Casey N. (1991) Feelings are part of caring. *Nurs Stand.* 5(48): 3.

Cecil R, editor. (1996) *The Anthropology of Pregnancy Loss.* Oxford: Berg.

Clark D. (2000) Death in Staithes. In: Dickenson D, Johnson M, Katz JS, editors. *Death, Dying and Bereavement.* London: Open University in association with Sage. pp. 4–9.

Corr CA, Nabe CM, Corr D. (1997) *Death and Dying, Life and Living.* 2nd ed. Pacific Grove, CA: Brooks/Cole.

Crookes PA. (1996) *Personal Bereavement and Registered General Nurses* [PhD thesis]. Hull: University of Hull.

Cutler L. (1998) Do intensive care nurses grieve for their patients? *Nurs Crit Care.* 3(4): 190–6.

Davis-Floyd R, Arvidson PS. (1997) *Intuition: the inside story; interdisciplinary perspectives.* London: Routledge.

Davis-Floyd R, Barclay L, Davies BA, *et al.* (2009) *Birth Models that Work.* Berkeley, CA: University of California Press.

Deery R. (2003) Engaging with clinical supervision in a community midwifery setting: an action research study [unpublished PhD thesis]. Sheffield: University of Sheffield.

Deery R and Kirkham M. (2007) Drained and dumped on: the generation and accumulation of emotional toxic waste in community midwifery. In: Kirkham M, editor. *Exploring the Dirty Side of Women's Health.* London: Routledge. pp. 63–74.

Deery R and Hunter B. (2010) Emotional work and relationships in midwifery. In: Kirkham M, editor. *The Midwife–Mother Relationship.* 2nd ed. Basingstoke: Macmillan. pp. 37–54.

Deery R, Hughes D, Kirkham M. (2010) *Tensions and Barriers to Improving Maternity Care: the story of a birth centre.* Oxford: Radcliffe.

Defey D. (1995) Helping healthcare staff deal with perinatal loss. *Infant Ment Health J.* 16(2): 102–11.

Denzin NK, Lincoln Y. (1998) *Collecting and Interpreting Qualitative Materials.* Thousand Oaks, CA: Sage.

Department of Health. (1993) *Changing Childbirth: report of the Expert Maternity Group.* London: HMSO.

———. (2004) *National Services Framework for Children, Young People and Maternity Services.* London: Department of Health.

———. (2007) *Maternity Matters: choice, access and continuity of care in a safe service.* London: DH.

Derbyshire F. (2000) Clinical supervision within midwifery. In: Kirkham M, editor. *Developments in the Supervision of Midwives.* Oxford: Books for Midwives. pp. 169–76.

Dickenson D, Johnson M, Katz J. (2000) *Death, Dying and Bereavement.* London: Sage.

Dixon NM. (1998) *Dialogue at Work: making talk developmental for people and organisations.* London: Lemos and Crane.

Doka KJ, editor. (2001) *Disenfranchised Grief: recognising hidden sorrow.* New York, NY: Lexington.

Edmondson A. (1999) Psychological safety and learning behaviour in work teams. *Adm Sci Q.* **44**: 350–83.

Edwards NP. (2005) *Birthing Autonomy.* London: Routledge.

Egan G. (1990) *The Skilled Helper: a systematic approach to effective helping.* 4th ed. Pacific Grove, CA: Brookes/Cole.

Engel GL. (1961) Is grief a disease? A challenge for medical research. *Psychosom Med.* **23**: 18–22.

Fahey-McCarthy E. (2003) Exploring theories of grief: personal reflection. *British Journal of Midwifery.* **11**(10): 595–603.

Fairtlough G, (1994) *Creative Compartments: a design for future organisation.* London: Adamantine Press.

Figley CR, Bride BE, Mazza N, editors (1997) *Death and Trauma: the traumatology of grieving.* Washington, DC: Taylor and Francis.

Finley L. (1998) Relexivity: an essential component for all research. *British Journal of Occupational Therapy.* **61**(10): 453–6.

Foster A. (1996) Perinatal bereavement support for families and midwives. *Midwives.* **109**(1303): 218–19.

Friedeberger J. (1996) *A Visible Wound: a healing journey through breast cancer.* Shaftesbury: Element.

Gardner JM. (1999) Perinatal death: uncovering the needs of midwives and nurses and exploring helpful interventions in the United States, England, and Japan. *J Transcult Nurs.* **10**(2): 120–30.

Garner H. (1996) *True Stories.* Melbourne: Text Publishing.

Garratt EF. (2010) *Survivors of Childhood Sexual Abuse and Midwifery Practice: CSA, birth and powerlessness.* Oxford: Radcliffe.

Gilham B. (2000) *The Research Interview.* London: Continuum.

Gillen P. (2007) *The Nature and Manifestations of Bullying in Midwifery* [PhD dissertation]. Belfast: University of Ulster.

Glaser BG, Strauss AL, (1967) *The Discovery of Grounded Theory.* London: Weidenfeld.

———. (1968) *A Time for Dying.* Chicago, IL: Aldine.

Greene R. (2002) Holocaust Survivors: a study in resilience. *J Gerontol Soc Work.* **37**: 3–18.

Hampden-Turner C. (1990) *Corporate Culture: from vicious to virtuous circles.* London: Hutchinson.

Hockey J. (1986) The human encounter with death: an anthropological approach [unpublished PhD thesis]. Durham: University of Durham.

——. (1989) Caring for the dying in acute hospitals. *Nurs Times.* **85**(39): 47–50.

Hockey J, Katz J, Small N. (2001) *Grief Mourning and Death Ritual.* Buckingham: Open University Press.

Hodnett ED, Gates S, Hofmyr GJ, *et al.* (2007) Continuous support for women during childbirth. Cochrane Database Syst Rev. 2011 2: CD003766.

Hollins Martin CJ, Bull P. (2008) Obedience and conformity in clinical practice. *British Journal of Midwifery.* **16**(8): 504–10.

Homer C, Brodie P, Leap N. (2001) *Establishing Models of Continuity of Midwifery Care in Australia: a resource for midwives.* Sydney: University of Technology, Sydney, Centre for Family Health and Midwifery.

——. (2008) *Midwifery Continuity of Care.* Sydney: Churchill Livingstone.

Hunter B, Deery R. (2009) *Emotions in Midwifery and Reproduction.* Basingstoke: Palgrave Macmillan.

Hunter B, Berg M, Lundgren I, *et al.* (2008) Relationships: the hidden threads in the tapestry of maternity care. *Midwifery.* **24**: 132–7.

Johns C. (2000) *Becoming a Reflective Practitioner.* Oxford: Blackwell Science.

——. (2002) *Guided Reflection: advancing practice.* Oxford: Blackwell.

——. (2004) *Being Mindful, Easing Suffering: reflections on palliative care.* London and Philadelphia, PA: Jessica Kingsley.

Jolly, J. (1987) *Missed Beginnings: death before life has been established.* London: Austen Cornish.

Jones O. (2000) Supervision in a midwife-managed birth centre. In: Kirkham M, editor. *Developments in the Supervision of Midwives.* Oxford: Books for Midwives. pp. 149–68.

Jordan B. (1993) *Birth in Four Cultures.* 4th ed. Prospect Heights, IL: Waveland Press.

Kaufman J. (1989) Intrapsychic dimensions of disenfranchised grief. In: Doka K, editor. *Disenfranchised Grief: recognising hidden sorrow.* Lexington, KY: Lexington Books. pp. 143–60.

Kenworthy D. (2004) The impact of loss on midwives: stillbirth the lived experience [unpublished PhD thesis]. Bradford: The University of Bradford.

Kirkham M. (1997) Stories and childbirth. In: Kirkham M, Perkins E, editors. *Reflections on Midwifery.* London: Bailliere Tindal. pp. 183–204.

——. (1999) The culture of midwifery in the NHS in England. *J Adv Nurs.* **30**(3): 732–9.

——, editor. (2003) *Birth Centres: a social model for maternity care.* Oxford: Elsevier Science.

——. (2009) *Review of Cases Cared for by Independent Midwives Where a Stillbirth or Neonatal Death Occurred.* Dundee: University of Dundee, Department of Nursing and Midwifery. Available at: www.dundee.ac.uk/nursingmidwifery/research/early-years-parenting (accessed 24 February 2011).

——, editor. (2010) *The Midwife–Mother Relationship.* 2nd ed. Basingstoke: Macmillan.

Kirkham M, Stapleton H, editors. (2001) *Informed Choice in Maternity Care: an evaluation of evidence based leaflets.* York: NHS Centre for Reviews and Dissemination.

Kirkham M, Morgan RK. (2006) *Why Midwives Return and their Subsequent Experience.* London: Department of Health and The University of Sheffield.

Kirkham M, Morgan RM, Davies C. (2006) *Why Midwives Stay.* London: Department of Health and The University of Sheffield.

Kirkham M, Stapleton H, Curtis P, *et al.* (2002) Stereotyping as a professional defence mechanism. *British Journal of Midwifery.* **10**(9): 509–13.

Klass D, Silverman PR, Nickman SL. (1996) *Continuing Bonds: new understandings of grief.* London: Taylor and Francis.

Klaus MH, Kennel JH. (1982) *Maternal-Infant Bonding.* St Louis, MO: Mosby.

Koch T. (1996) *Implementation of a Hermeneutic Enquiry in Nursing: philosophy, rigour and representation.* Cited in: Smith BA. (1999) Clinical scholarship: ethical and methodologic benefits of using a reflexive journal in hermeneutic-phenomenologic research. *Image J Nurs Sch.* **31**(4): 359–63.

Kubler-Ross E. (1970) *On Death and Dying.* London: Tavistock.

Lamers WM. (1997) How patient deaths affect health professionals: a plea for more open communication. *J Pain Palliat Care Pharmacother.* **5**(3): 59–71.

Laungani P. (1995) Patterns of bereavement in Indian British society. *Bereave Care.* **14**(1): 5–7.

Lawton J. (2000) *The Dying Process.* London: Routledge.

Leap N. (1997) Making sense of 'horizontal violence' in midwifery. *British Journal of Midwifery.* **5**(11): 689.

——. (2010) The less we do the more we give. In: Kirkham M, editor. *The Midwife–Mother Relationship.* 2nd ed. Basingstoke: Macmillan. pp. 17–36.

Lindemann E. (1944) Symptomatology and management of acute grief. *Am J Psychiatry.* **101**: 141–8.

Lomas P. (2005) *Cultivating Intuition.* 2nd ed. London: Whurr.

Lovell H. (1986) Mothers' reactions to perinatal death. *Nurs Times.* **12**: 40–4.

McCourt C, Stevens T. (2009) Relationship and reciprocity in caseload midwifery. In: Hunter B, Deery R, editors. *Emotions in Midwifery and Reproduction.* Basingstoke: Palgrave. pp.17–35.

McCracken E. (2009) *An Exact Replica of a Figment of My Imagination.* London: Jonathan Cape.

Machin L. (2009) *Working with Loss and Grief.* London: Sage.

McVicar A. (2003) Workplace stress in nursing: a literature review. *J Adv Nurs.* **44**(6): 633–42.

Magowan B., Owen P. and Drife J. (2009) *Clinical Obstetrics and Gynaecology.* Second ed. London: Saunders, Elsevier. p. 387.

Malby R, Pattison S. (1999) *Living Values in the NHS: stories from the NHS's 50th year.* London: King's Fund.

Mander R. (1996) The childfree midwife: the significance of personal experience of childbearing. *Midwives.* **109**(1302): 186–8.

——. (2001) The midwife's ultimate paradox: a UK-based study of the death of a mother. *Midwifery.* **17**(4): 248–59.

——. (2006) *Loss and Bereavement in Childbearing.* 2nd ed. London: Routledge.

Marmot M. (2004) *Status Syndrome.* London: Bloomsbury.

Marris P. (1974) *Loss and Change.* London: Routledge.

——. (1996) *The Politics of Uncertainty: attachment in private and public life.* London: Routledge.

Menzies Lyth I. (1988) *Containing Anxiety in Institutions: selected essays Volume 1.* London: Free Association Books.

Minardi HA, Riley MJ. (1997) *Communication in Healthcare: a skills-based approach.* Oxford: Butterworth-Heinemann.

Morell CM. (1994) *Unwomanly Conduct: the challenges of intentional childlessness.* London: Routledge.

Moustakas C. (1994) *Phenomenological Research Methods.* London: Sage.

NICE (National Institute for Health and Clinical Excellence). (2007) Antenatal and Postnatal Mental Health: clinical management and service guidance. NICE guideline 45. London: NIHCE. http://guidance.nice.org.uk/nicemedia/live/11004/30433/30433.pdf (accessed 24 February 2011).

——. (2010) *Clarification statement on stillbirth recommendation in pregnancy-related guidance: NICE guideline 45.* London: NIHCE. www.nice.org.uk/CG045

Nuland SB. (1994) *How We Die.* London: Chatto and Windus.

NMC (Nursing and Midwifery Council). (2008) *The Code: standards of conduct, performance and ethics for nurses and midwives.* London: NMC.

Olafsdottir OA, Kirkham M. (2009) Narrative time: stories, childbirth and midwifery. In: McCourt C, editor. *Childbirth, Midwifery and Concepts of Time.* Oxford: Berghahn Books. pp. 167–83.

Orbach S. (1994) *What's Really Going on Here?* London: Virago.

Oxford Dictionary. 2003 Available at: www.askoxford.com (accessed 28 February 2011).

Parkes CM. (1996) *Bereavement: studies of grief in adult life.* 3rd ed. Harmondsworth: Penguin.

——. (1998) Traditional models and theories of grief. *Bereave Care.* **17**(2): 21–3.

——. (2002) Grief: lessons from the past, visions for the future. *Death Stud.* **26**(5): 367–85.

——. (2006) *Love and Loss: the roots of grief and its complications.* London: Routledge.

Parkes CM, Weiss RS. (1983) *Recovery from Bereavement.* New York, NY: Basic Books.

Payne N. (2001) Occupational stressors and coping as determinants of burnout in female hospice nurses. *J Adv Nurs.* **33**(3): 396–405.

Perkins BB. (2004) *The Medical Delivery Business.* New Brunswick, NJ: Rutgers University Press.

Portch M. (1995) *Communications and Interpersonal Skills.* London: Hodder and Stoughton Educational Publications.

Price DM, Murphy PA. (1985) Emotional depletion in critical care staff. *J Neurosurg Nurs.* **17**(2): 114–18.

Prior L. (2000) The social distribution of sentiments. In: Dickenson D, Johnson M, Katz JS, editors. *Death, Dying, and Bereavement.* London: Sage. pp. 332–7.

Purtilo R, Haddad A. (1996) *Health Professional and Patient Interaction.* 5th ed. Philadelphia, PA: WB Saunders.

Raphael B. (1996) *The Anatomy of Bereavement.* London: Routledge.

Rashotte J, Fothergill-Bourbonnais F, Chamberlain M. (1997) Paediatric intensive care nurses and their grief experiences: a phenomenological study. *Heart Lung.* **26**(5): 372–86.

RCM (Royal College of Midwives). (1996) *In Place of Fear: recognising and confronting the problem of bullying in midwifery.* London: RCM.

RCM, RCN (Royal College of Nursing). (2000) *Collaborative Study: experiences of returning to practice.* London: The Stationery Office.

Reynolds JL. (1997) Post traumatic stress disorder after childbirth: the phenomenon of traumatic birth. *CMAJ.* **156**(6): 831–5.

Riches G, Dawson P. (2000) *An Intimate Loneliness: supporting the bereaved parents and siblings.* Buckingham: Open University Press.

Robinson J. (2003) Professional fear: a barrier to consent. *British Journal of Midwifery.* **11**(12): 719.

Rosenberg MB. (2003) *Nonviolent Communication: a language for life.* Encinitas, CA: Puddle Dancer Press.

Rothman KB. (1996) Women, providers and control. *J Obstet Gynecol Neonatal Nurs.* **25**(3): 253–6.

Sandall J. (1997) Midwives' burnout and continuity of care. *British Journal of Midwifery.* **5**(2): 106–11.

Sarton M. (1980) *Writings on Writing.* London: Women's Press.

Saunders JM, Valente SM. (1994) Nurses' Grief. *Cancer Nurs.* **17**(4): 318–25.

Savage J. (1995) *Nursing Intimacy: an ethnographic approach to nurse–patient interaction.* London: Scutari.

Simkin P. (1996) The experience of maternity in a woman's life. *J Obstet Gynecol Neonatal Nurs.* **25**(3) 247–52.

Speckard A. (1997) Traumatic death in pregnancy: the significance of meaning and attachment. In: Fidgley CR, Bride BE, Mazza N, editors. *Death and Trauma: the traumatology of grieving.* Washington, DC: Taylor and Francis. pp. 67–100.

Spencer L. (1994) How do nurses deal with their own grief when a patient dies on an intensive care unit, and what help can be given to enable them to overcome their grief effectively? *J Adv Nurs.* **19**: 1141–50.

Staudacher C. (1987) *Beyond Grief: a guide for recovering from the death of a loved one.* Oakland, CA: New Harbour.

Stevens TA. (2003) *Midwife to Mid Wif: a study of case load midwifery* [PhD thesis]. London: Thames Valley University.

Stroebe M, Schut H. (1999) The dual process model of coping with bereavement: rationale and description. *Death Stud.* **23**(3): 197–224.

Stroebe W, Stroebe M. (1987) *Bereavement and Health.* Cambridge: Cambridge University Press.

Symon A, Winter C, Inkster M, *et al.* (2009) Outcomes for births booked under the care of an independent midwife and births in NHS maternity units: a matched comparison study. *BMJ.* **338**: B2060.

Taylor M. (2010) The midwife as container. In: Kirkham M, editor. *The Midwife–Mother Relationship.* 2nd ed. Basingstoke: Macmillan. pp. 232–49.

Taylor SE. (2002) *The Tending Instinct.* New York: Henry Holt.

Thomas SP. (1998) *Transforming Nurses' Anger and Pain.* New York, NY: Springer.

Too S. (1995) Grief counselling following stillbirth. *Midwives.* **8**(1291): 260–2.

Vadeboncoeur H. (2010) *Birthing Normally after a Caesarean or Two: a guide for pregnant women; exploring reasons and practicalities for VBAC.* Chester le Street: Fresh Heart.

Wakefield A. (2000) Nurses' responses to death and dying: a need for relentless self-care. *Int J Palliat Nurs.* **6**(5): 245–50.

Waldenstrom U. (2003) Women's memories of childbirth at two months and one year after the birth. *Birth.* **30**(4): 248–54.

Walter T. (1999) *On Bereavement: the culture of grief.* Buckingham: Open University Press.

Weber M. (1968) *On Charisma and Institution Building.* Eisenstadt SN, editor. Chicago, IL: University of Chicago Press.

Weinberg N. (1995) Does apologizing help? The role of self-blame and making amends in recovery from bereavement. *Health Soc Work.* **20**(4): 194–300.

Weston R, Martin T, Anderson Y. (1998) *Loss and Bereavement: managing change.* Oxford: Blackwell Science.

Wilde V. (1992) Controversial hypotheses on the relationship between researcher and informant in qualitative research. *J Adv Nurs.* **17**: 234–42.

Wood L, Quenby S. (2010) Exploring pregnancy following a pre-term birth or pregnancy loss. *British Journal of Midwifery.* **18**(6): 350–6.

Worden JW. (2003) *Grief Counselling and Grief Therapy: a handbook for the mental health practitioner.* 3rd ed. New York: Springer.

Wright L. (1998) Sudden infant death: how do health visitors cope? *Community Pract.* **71**(3): 103–5.

Index

anger
>defusing 93, 97, 151
>from families 92
>transference of 98
>unresolved 23–4

anxiety, defences against 143, 145, 147
apology 82, 92, 100, 108, 116, 118, 123
assertiveness 31–3, 59
attachment behaviour 111
attachment theory 10
authority 152
autonomy
>of IMs 121, 143
>loss of 137, 157
>maternal 125–6

beliefs, personal 23, 100, 113–14
bereavement
>as activity 12
>and feelings of failure 81–2
>and intuitive knowing 41
>and memories 44
>and miscarriage 11
>positive aspects of 21
>simultaneous of midwife and client 32
>stages of 9–10
bereavement empathy 65–6
Bereavement Support Midwives 1
birth centres 146–7, 154, 156–7
bitterness 113–14, 153
blame
>and apology 108
>attributing 114
>from colleagues 91, 99–103
>compulsive 140
>as coping mechanism 70
>culture of 152–3
>for mother 128–9

and relations between midwives 117
of self, *see* self-blame
body language 3, 30–1, 36, 75, 78, 92–3, 119

caesarean 77, 121, 124–5, 127
care
>continuity of 51, 55, 59, 77, 121, 124,
>>133, 137, 141, 154
>philosophy of 125
>reciprocal 70
>standardising 152, 157
care-eliciting behaviour 111
care-giving, security in 10
childbirth, image of 24
clinical supervision, *see* midwives,
>supervision of
communication
>defensive 55
>fragmentation of 108–9
>nonviolent, *see* Nonviolent
>>Communication
confidentiality 6, 99, 121, 138, 147
conflict, internalised 86
congruence 36, 75, 110
connectedness 13, 42, 75
coping strategies 13–15, 30–1, 34, 136–7,
>150, 158
coroners 37, 94, 122–3
counselling 100, 110, 116–17, 130, 139,
>147, 159
culpability 17, 43, 87, 91–4, 96, 139
cultural change 147–8, 153–4, 160

death
>anticipated 42
>and healthcare professionals 13–15, 138
>in hospital 8–9
>images of 28, 45